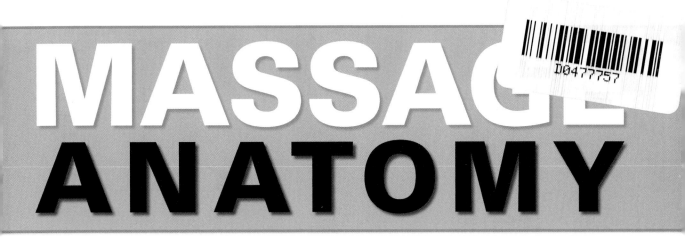

MASSAGE
ANATOMY

D0477757

General Disclaimer

The contents of this book are intended to provide useful information to the general public. All materials, including texts, graphics, and images, are for informational purposes only and are not a substitute for medical diagnosis, advice, or treatment for specific medical conditions. All readers should seek expert medical care and consult their own physicians before commencing any exercise program or for any general or specific health issues. The author and publishers do not recommend or endorse specific treatments, procedures, advice, or other information found in this book and specifically disclaim all responsibility for any and all liability, loss, or risk, personal or otherwise, which is incurred as a consequence, directly or indirectly, of the use or application of any of the material in this publication.

Thunder Bay Press
An imprint of the Baker & Taylor Publishing Group
10350 Barnes Canyon Road, San Diego, CA 92121
www.thunderbaybooks.com

THUNDER BAY
P · R · E · S · S

Copyright © Moseley Road Inc. 2009

Copyright under International, Pan American, and Universal Copyright Conventions. All rights reserved. No part of this book may be reproduced or transmitted in any form or by any means, electronic or mechanical, including photocopying, recording, or by any information storage-and-retrieval system, without written permission from the copyright holder. Brief passages (not to exceed 1,000 words) may be quoted for reviews.

"Thunder Bay" is a registered trademark of Baker & Taylor. All rights reserved.

All notations of errors or omissions should be addressed to Thunder Bay Press, Editorial Department, at the above address. All other correspondence (author inquiries, permissions) concerning the content of this book should be addressed to Moseley Road, Inc., 129 Main Street, Irvington, NY 10533. www.moseleyroad.com.

ISBN-13: 978-1-60710-014-0
ISBN-10: 1-60710-014-2

Printed in Canada

1 2 3 4 5 13 12 11 10 09

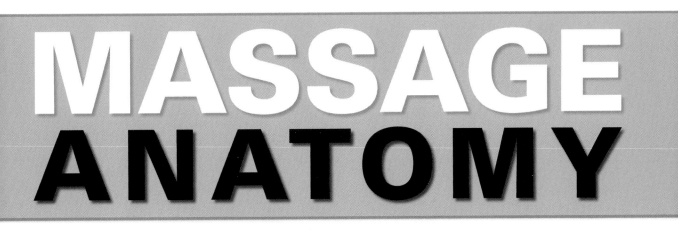

MASSAGE ANATOMY

A Comprehensive Guide

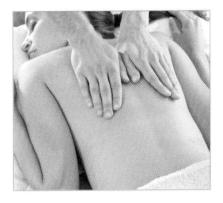

Dr. Abby Ellsworth
and Peggy Altman

THUNDER BAY
P · R · E · S · S

San Diego, California

CONTENTS

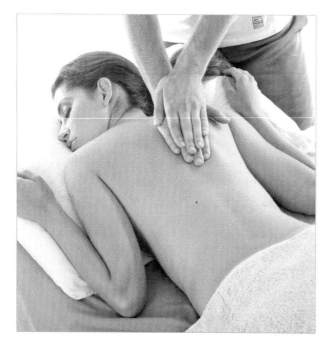

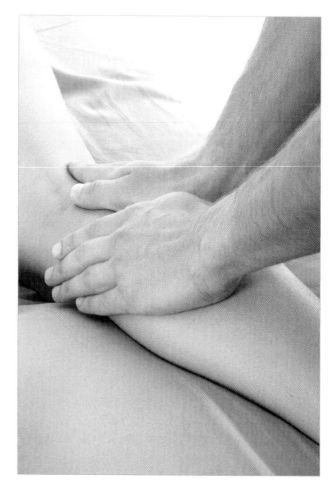

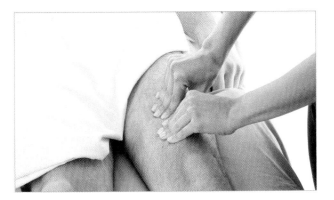

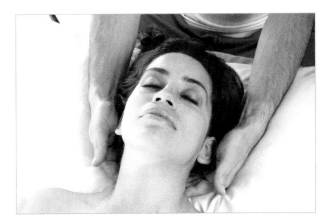

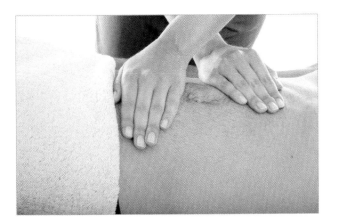

INTRODUCTION

Who doesn't love a good massage? Unfortunately, booking an appointment with a professional massage therapist requires time and expense. But what if you had the know-how to give (or receive) a massage at home that was almost as good as one that you would receive from a professional?

That's where MASSAGE ANATOMY comes in. This detailed guide to massage provides you with everything you need give a massage in your home.

The massage demonstrated on the following pages is a basic Swedish massage. It incorporates a series of hand strokes, kneading movements, and "friction" (more about that later) to work the muscles. Our massage is about relaxing tense muscles, improving the range of motion of joints, stress relief, and enhancing circulation.

MASSAGE ANATOMY also offers you flexibility. When you don't have time for a full-body massage, you can pick and choose from the

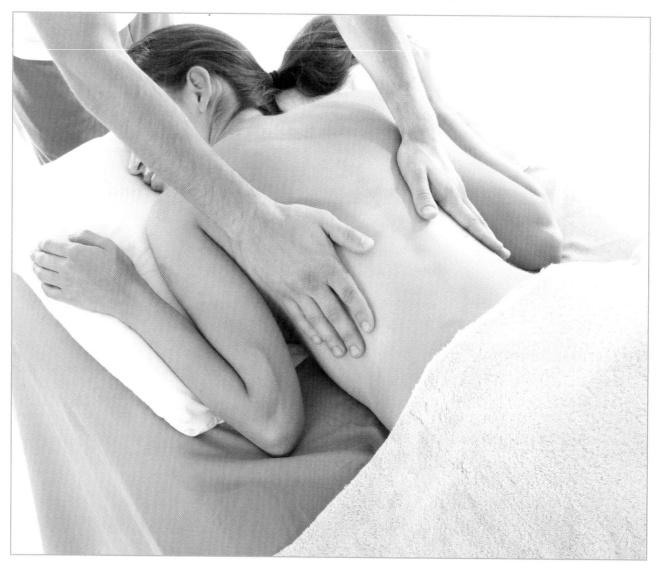

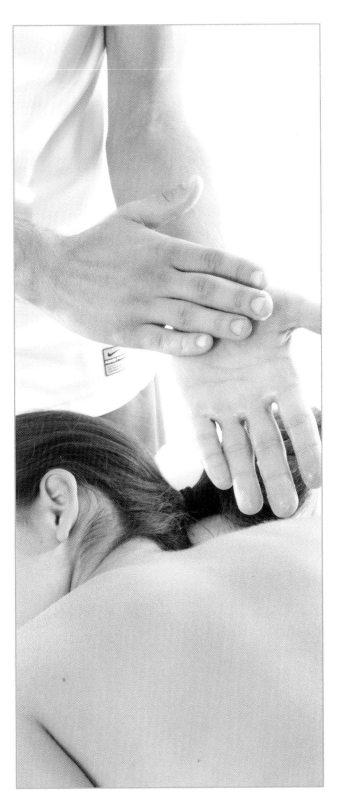

WHAT IT'S GOOD FOR

From anxiety to tension headaches, massage therapy has been shown to provide relief for a whole host of conditions. Here are just a few. (Keep in mind that some of these disorders require professional massage therapy to show improvement.)

- Allergies
- Anxiety and stress
- Arthritis (osteoarthritis and rheumatoid)
- Asthma
- Bronchitis
- Carpal tunnel syndrome
- Chronic back pain
- Depression
- Fibromyalgia
- Insomnia
- Lower-back pain
- Shoulder pain
- Sinusitis
- Sports injuries
- Tension headaches

techniques to create a shorter massage. For instance, perhaps your spouse has come home from a long day on her feet. You could treat her to a foot massage using the instructions from this book. Or you may choose to focus on the head and neck of a friend suffering from a tension headache.

MASSAGE ANATOMY opens with a discussion of the basics of massage. We include expert advice about how to set up a massage space in your home, what items you'll want to have on hand,

INTRODUCTION (CONTINUED)

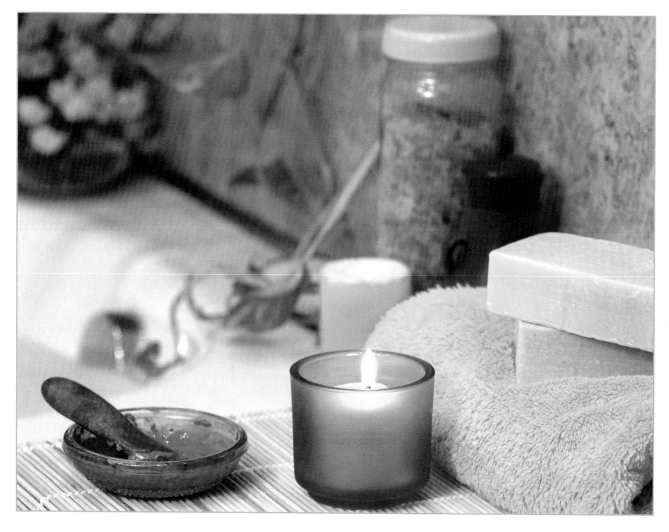

how to set the mood, and even which oils work best. From there, the book proceeds to the massage itself, starting with the back, moving to the legs, feet, abs and chest, and ending with a soothing face and head massage that will rival any you might receive from a professional massage therapist.

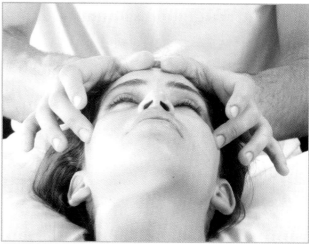

At every step of the way, we provide detailed and labeled anatomical illustrations that allow you to "see" the muscles you're working on as well as the other structures, such as bones, that you need to be aware of as you give your massage. You'll also find "Caution" boxes that alert you to important information, such as when not to massage a particular part of the body, and "Massage Tips" sidebars that explain more about a particular stroke.

At the back of the book are a series of massage programs, ideas for shorter massage sequences when you don't have time to offer a total-body massage, a glossary of frequently used massage terms, and finally, a page of resources, including retailers that sell oils, tables, and other massage-related supplies.

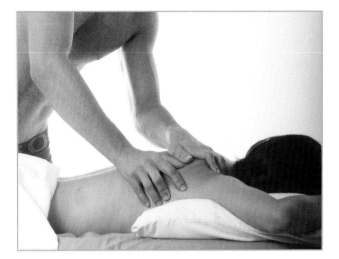

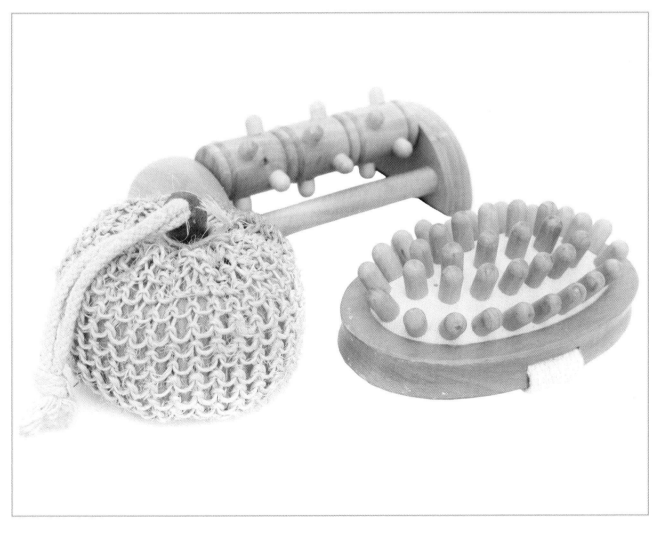

BASICS

The first step to giving a good massage is creating a relaxed and calm atmosphere. So shoo the kids and move the pet bird to another room. Turn off the television.

Next close the shades and dim the lights or, if you prefer, light some candles. Unscented candles are the best bet if you're using scented massage oil. Clashing scents can be bothersome for the person you're massaging; in fact,

he or she may be allergic. The same goes for you: avoid strong-smelling perfumes or colognes. On the other hand, the person you're massaging may enjoy scented candles or even incense, so be sure to ask.

The room temperature should be comfortable for the person receiving the massage, as he or she will be nude (although covered by a sheet).

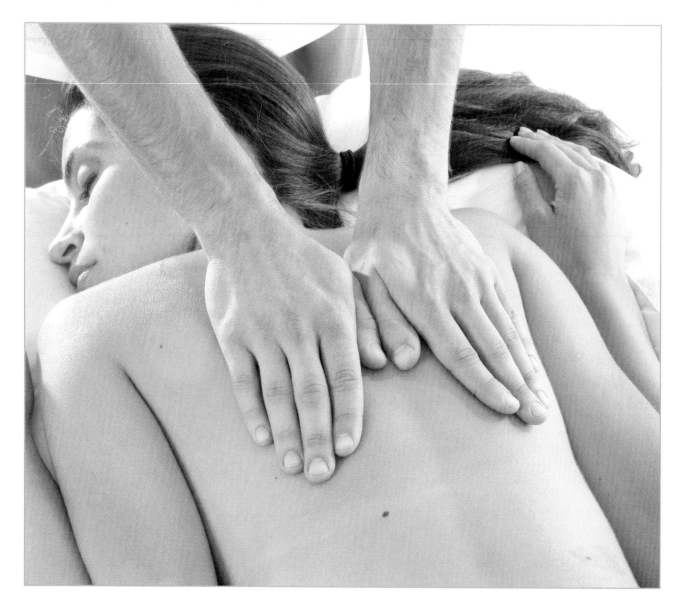

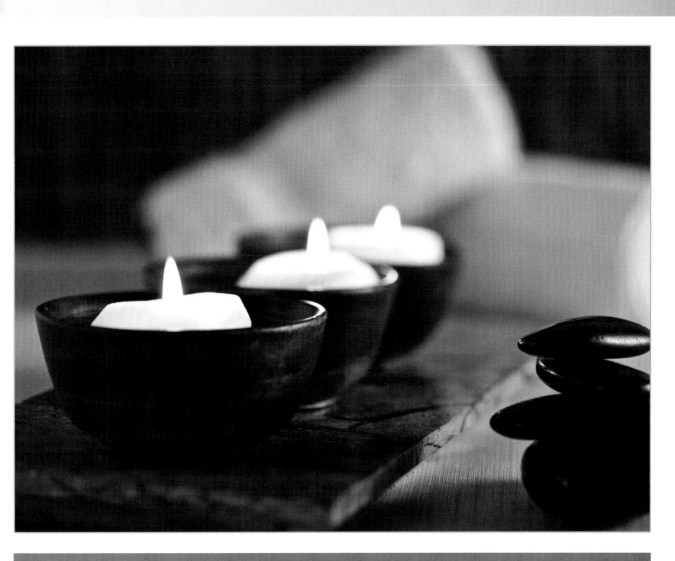

PREPARING THE TABLE

In addition to creating a pleasant atmosphere, you will need to have some items on hand before you start a massage. Once you have a table (or other sturdy surface), you'll need several sheets: one to cover its surface and another to cover the person you're massaging. Cotton sheets are best, but don't use your most expensive set, as they'll end up stained with oil. If possible, choose patterned sheets over solid colors, as they'll hide any oil stains better.

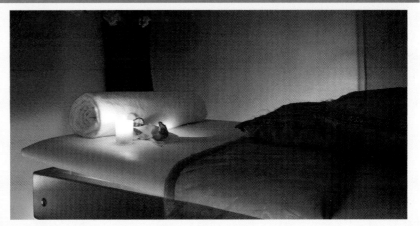

BASICS (CONTINUED)

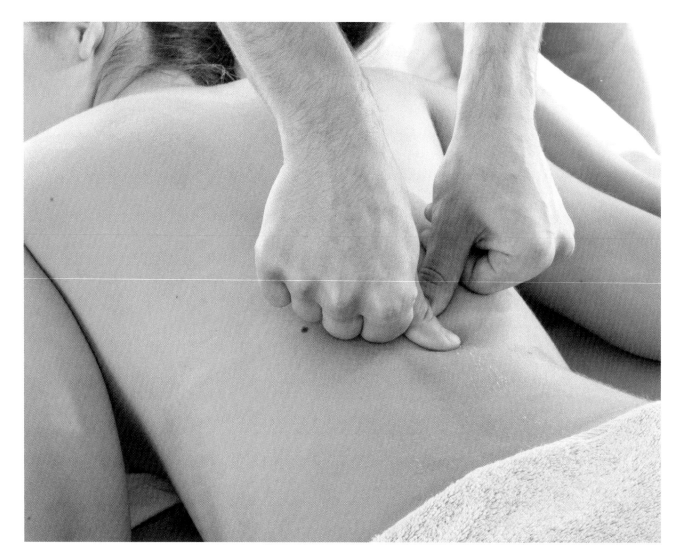

Massage oil is a must; it allows your hands to glide over your subject's skin. Among the most popular oils for massage are sweet almond oil (don't use in the case of nut allergies), apricot kernel oil, and jojoba oil (which is actually a liquid wax). You'll also need a handy spot to set the oil.

What you wear is up to you, with one exception: long sleeves are liable to get stained by the oil and could tickle the person you're massaging, so opt for short sleeves.

When determining where to give a massage, there are a few factors to keep in mind. First, the surface should be comfortable for the massage giver and receiver. For the giver, that means an appropriate height. Here's a way to gauge what that is: Stand straight with your hands at your sides. Make a fist with both hands and see where the first set of knuckles are. That's how high your table should be. If the table is too high or too low, you risk straining and ending up with aches and pains.

WITH AND AGAINST THE MUSCLE GRAIN

Muscle fibers grow in an organized way, forming the muscle's "grain," in much the same way that wood has a grain. Throughout this book, you'll see references to massaging with and against the grain of a particular muscle. Massaging against the grain of a muscle can reduce scar tissue and increase flexibility.

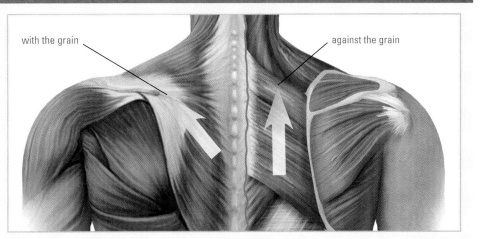

with the grain

against the grain

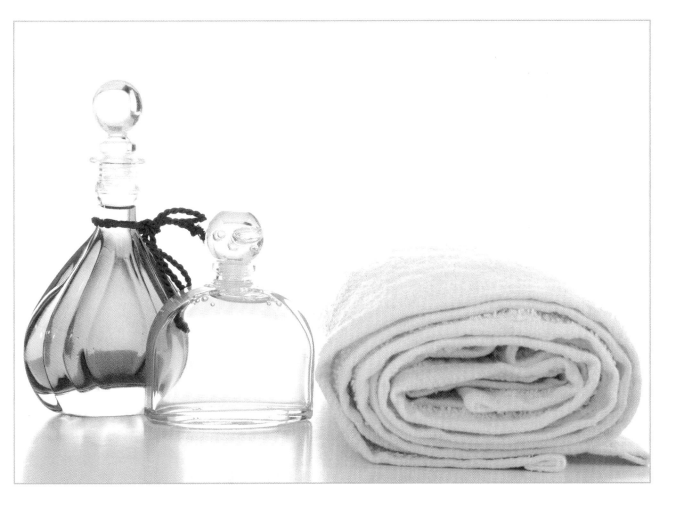

BASICS (CONTINUED)

When you're giving a massage at home, there are a few rules of thumb to consider. For instance, both you and the person receiving the massage should be comfortable at all times. Before you begin, ask your subject to let you know if he or she becomes uncomfortable at any point for any reason. Make sure you don't strain to reach your subject. Always stand within easy reach of the person you're massaging.

Massage should never cause pain! If it does, stop what you're doing immediately.

Massage is in large part about touch. Always strive to keep at least one hand in contact with the person you're massaging at all times. It's unpleasant for the person being massaged to suddenly feel "abandoned" by the massager. This will require that you pay attention—especially during transitions from one body part to another. You may be surprised to find how mindful you'll need to be!

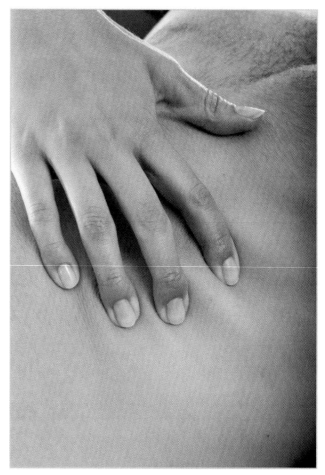

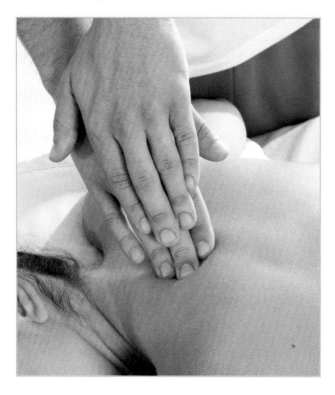

MASSAGE RULES OF THUMB

- Both you and the person you're massaging should always be comfortable.

- Ask the person you're massaging to speak up if something doesn't feel good or if he feels too cold or too warm.

- Massage should never hurt; if it does, stop.

- Never press on the spine or massage it directly.

- If the person you're massaging is feeling ticklish, go more slowly and more deeply.

- Don't abruptly take your hands off the person you're massaging. Always try to keep at least one hand on him.

CHOOSING A SURFACE

The height of the massage surface is important for the person giving the massage. Too high or low and the massager risks straining his or her own muscles and joints.

The height guidelines on page 12 are appropriate for moderate-pressure Swedish massage. If you want to apply less pressure, choose a higher table; for more pressure, choose a lower table.

Massaging someone on a bed is fine as long as the person can keep his or her back straight. A firm mattress or futon is best; too-soft mattresses don't provide enough support.

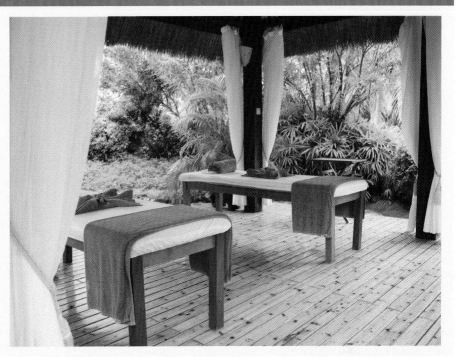

MORE ABOUT MASSAGE OILS

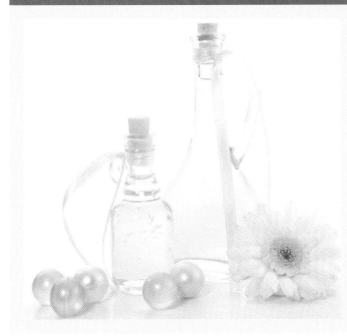

It's vital to use an oil when you give a massage because your hands need to slide and glide over the person's skin. In a pinch, you can use lotion. However, it doesn't provide much "slip," and so you'll end up using a lot of it.

Almost any vegetable oil can work for a massage, but be mindful of scent: Use olive oil and you'll end up smelling like a salad. The best bet is an oil sold specifically for massage; it may seem expensive, but in the long run, you'll use less of it compared to heavier oils that don't spread as far.

After a massage, be sure to wash the sheets immediately. Doing so will increase the chances that any oil on the sheets will wash out. And one last important note: oils are flammable; always keep candles or any other open flame away from them and the sheets.

BASICS (CONTINUED)

There are some parts of the body that should not be massaged, usually because arteries, nerves, organs, or veins are close to the surface of the skin. These areas—called endangerment zones—should be avoided in home massage.

Some examples of endangerment zones on the body include the eye sockets, the spine, the throat, the xiphoid process (the tip of the sternum), the soft area between the last rib and the hip bone, the knee, and on the ulnar nerve where it passes over the elbow.

Throughout this book, we note endangerment zones in the text and in "Caution" boxes.

In addition, people with certain conditions and ailments should not receive a home massage. For instance, a pregnant woman should be massaged only by a professional massage therapist; the same is true for anyone suffering from advanced osteoporosis.

If you feel that you're coming down with a cold or the flu, avoid getting—or giving—a massage. Someone with varicose veins can receive a massage, but not directly on the veins.

MASSAGE CONTRAINDICATIONS

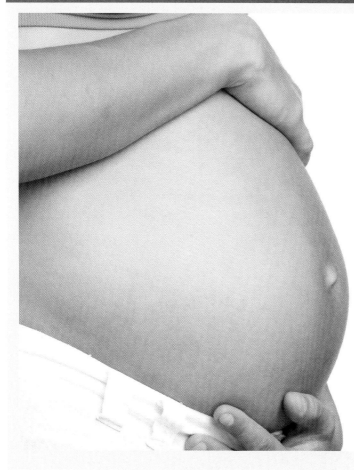

- Pregnant women should see a professional massage therapist rather than having one at home. In addition, people suffering from the following conditions should not receive a massage. If you have any chronic illness or are unsure, check with your own physician before having a massage.

- Advanced osteoporosis. Light massage is okay in the case of mild osteoporosis.

- Broken bones (avoid only the affected area)

- Cancer

- Cold or flu

- Fever

- Recent or healing wounds (avoid only the affected area)

- Skin rashes or blisters (avoid only the affected area). Some rashes and fungal infections (such as athlete's foot) can be spread by massage.

- Varicose veins

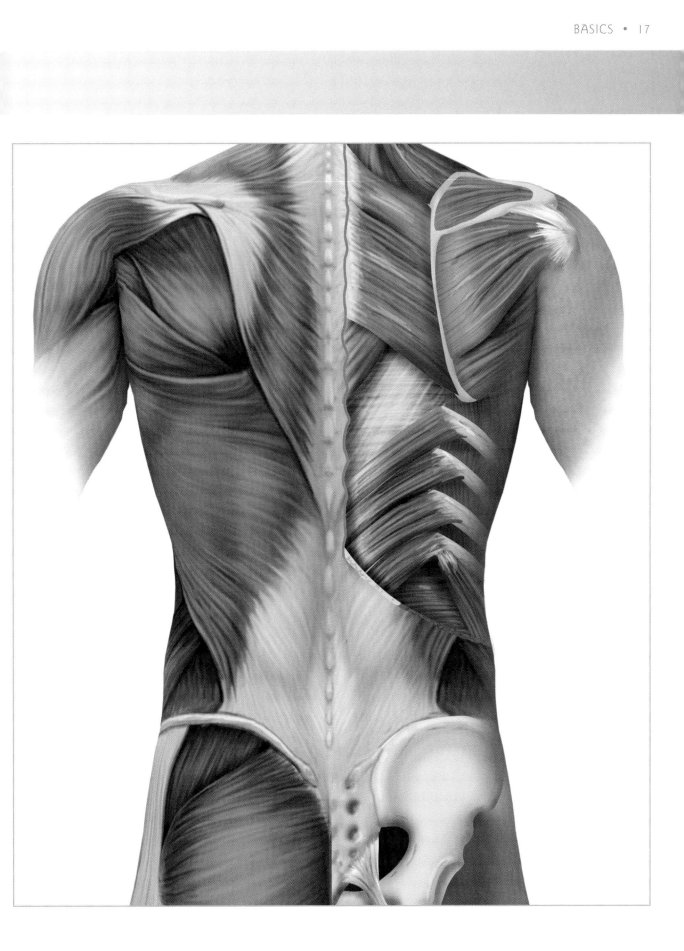

① UPPER BODY: BACK

Our full-body massage begins with the back. If the last back massage you gave (or received) consisted of a few quick squeezes along the shoulders, you're in for a delightful education.

Our directions begin with some light touches—effleurage—all over your subject's back. Then you will gradually work your way toward your subject's hips.

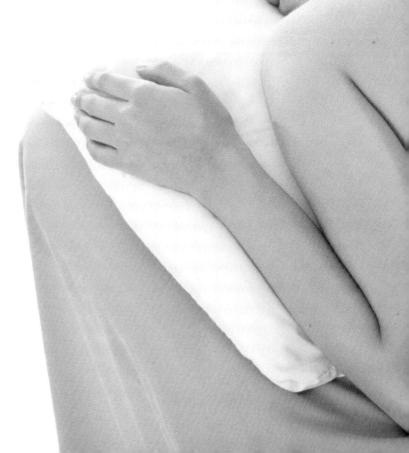

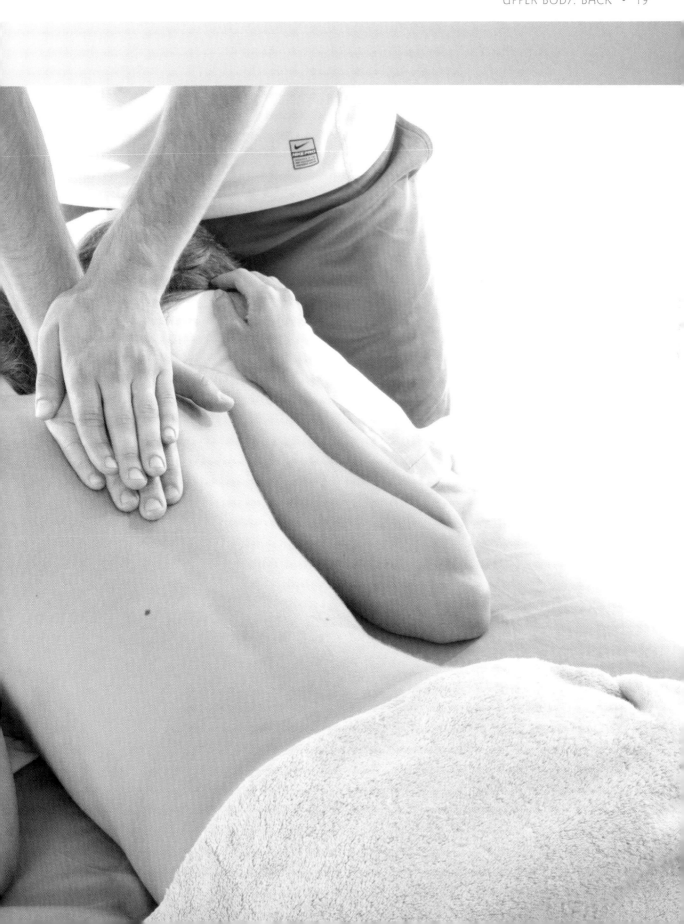

THE BACK

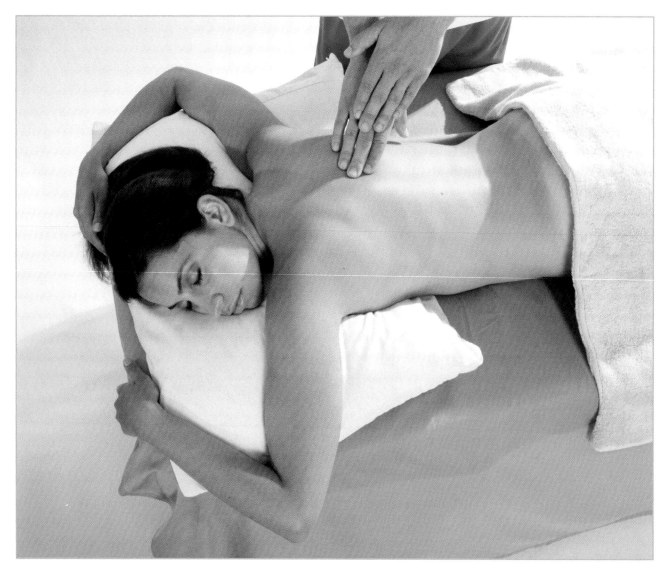

Your aching back! So much conspires to cause it pain: stress, poor posture while standing and sitting at a computer, pulling heavy suitcases, lifting heavy objects, driving, carrying heavy handbags, wearing high heels, and even walking around in flip-flops are all culprits. This portion of the massage will help your subject relax, unwind, and bring some welcome relief for her aching back muscles.

A word of caution: The spine is an endangerment area; never press directly on it.

CAUTION

AVOID MASSAGING YOUR SUBJECT'S BACK IF:

• She suffers from any acute back problems.

• She is experiencing shooting back pain.

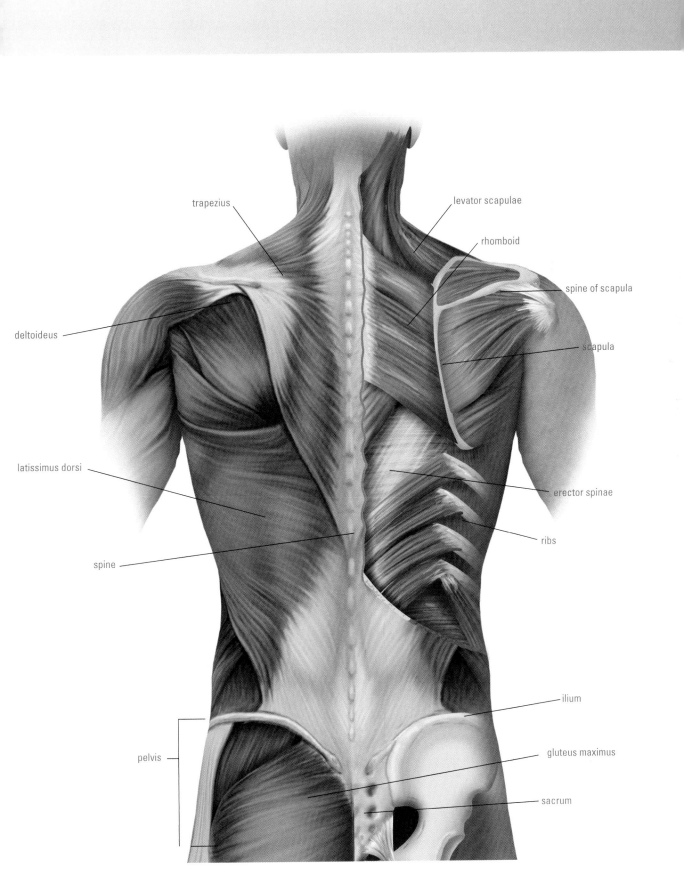

trapezius

levator scapulae

rhomboid

spine of scapula

deltoideus

scapula

latissimus dorsi

erector spinae

spine

ribs

pelvis

ilium

gluteus maximus

sacrum

THE BACK (CONTINUED)

A massage always starts with effleurage, or the initial touch. Its purpose is to warm the skin and get the blood flowing.

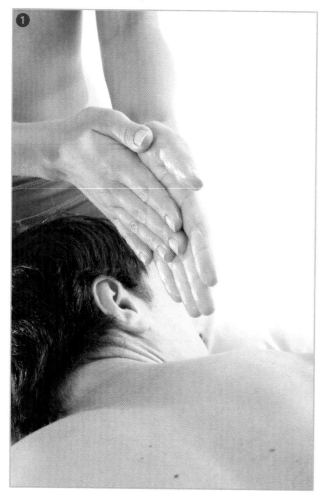

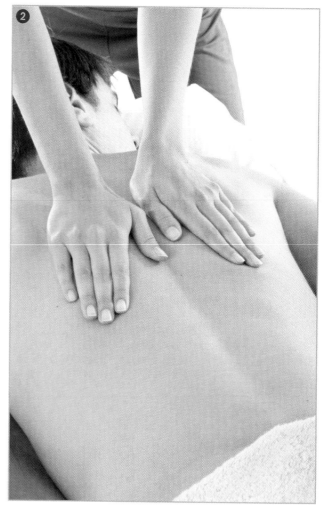

❶ To begin, stand in front of one of your subject's shoulders. Pour a little oil in the palm of your hand and rub your hands together to warm your hands and the oil. Then gently and slowly place your hands on your subject.

❷ Next, place each of your palms on either side of your subject's spine at the top of his shoulders. Make sure the entire surface of both palms is—and remains—in contact with the skin.

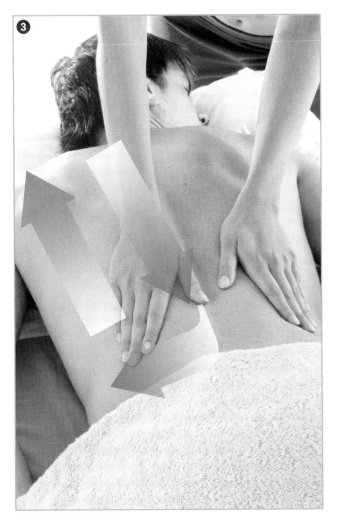

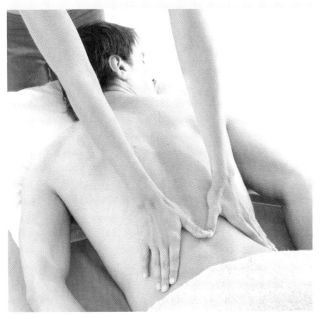

WATCH YOUR HANDS

When you give a massage, make sure to keep a gentle angle between your arm and hand. When you press straight down, you jam your wrists and shoulders.

CAUTION

The spine is an endangerment zone—never place direct pressure on it.

3 While maintaining constant contact with his skin, run your hands from the top of your subject's shoulders to the top of his sacrum, over to his hips, and then up his sides to his shoulders again. Move both hands together in the same direction or in opposite directions.

THE BACK (CONTINUED)

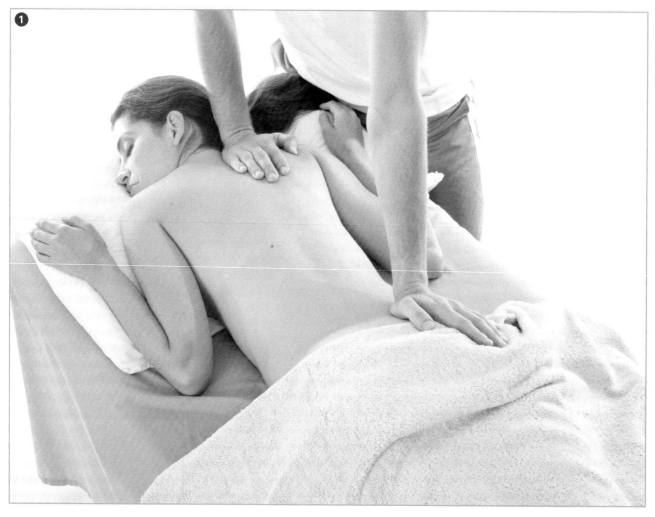

❶ Once you've finished with the effleurage strokes, place one of your hands over your subject's shoulder blade. Place the heel of your other hand against your subject's ilium and gently stretch that side of your subject's back by pulling your hands in opposite directions. Repeat on the other side.

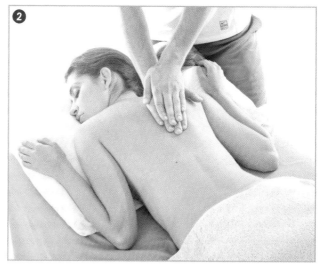

❷–❹ Next, place one hand atop the other and press into your subject's back, from the shoulder to the sacral area. Repeat on the other side of her spine.

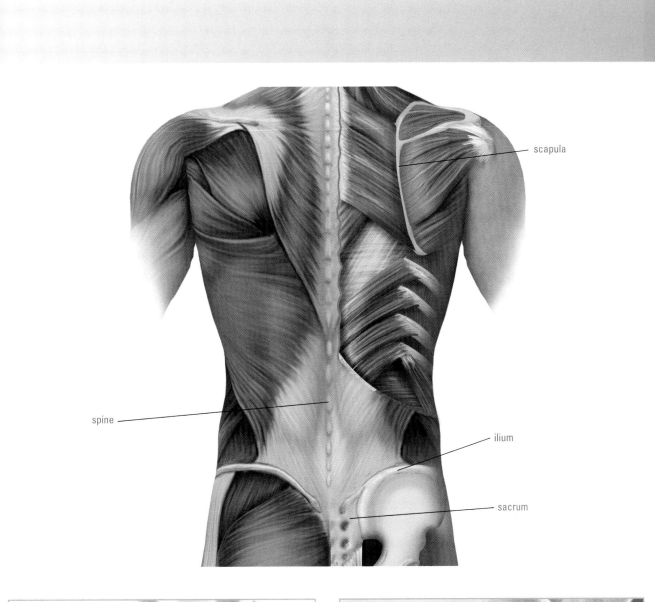

scapula

spine

ilium

sacrum

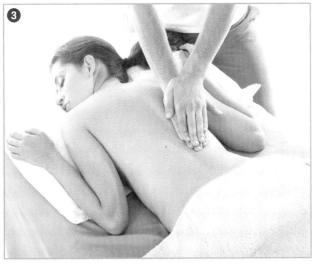

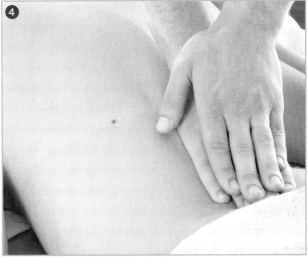

THE BACK (CONTINUED)

①–③ Place the meaty part of your forearm on your subject's upper back—since your forearm has more surface area than your hands, it creates a more satisfying sensation. Keep your wrist relaxed, and be sure to not jam your shoulder. Slide and glide your way down her back. Gently slide your forearm off her back when you get to her waist.

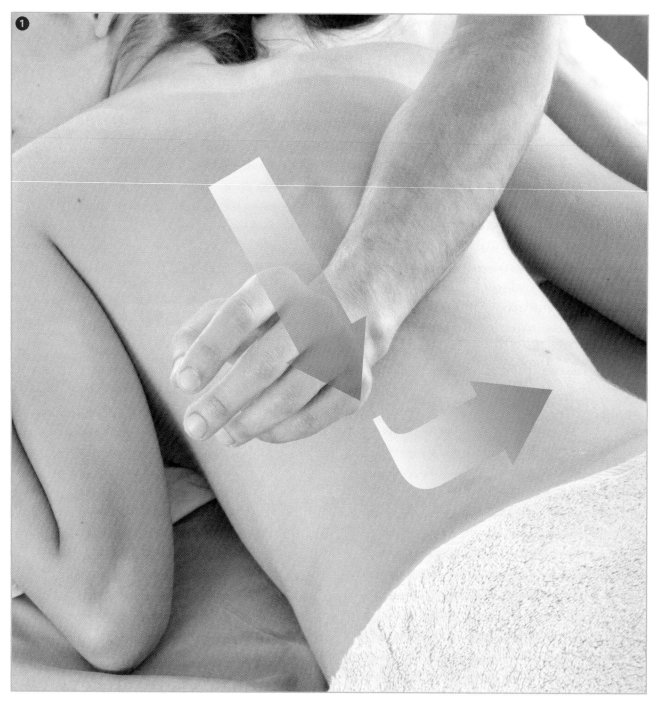

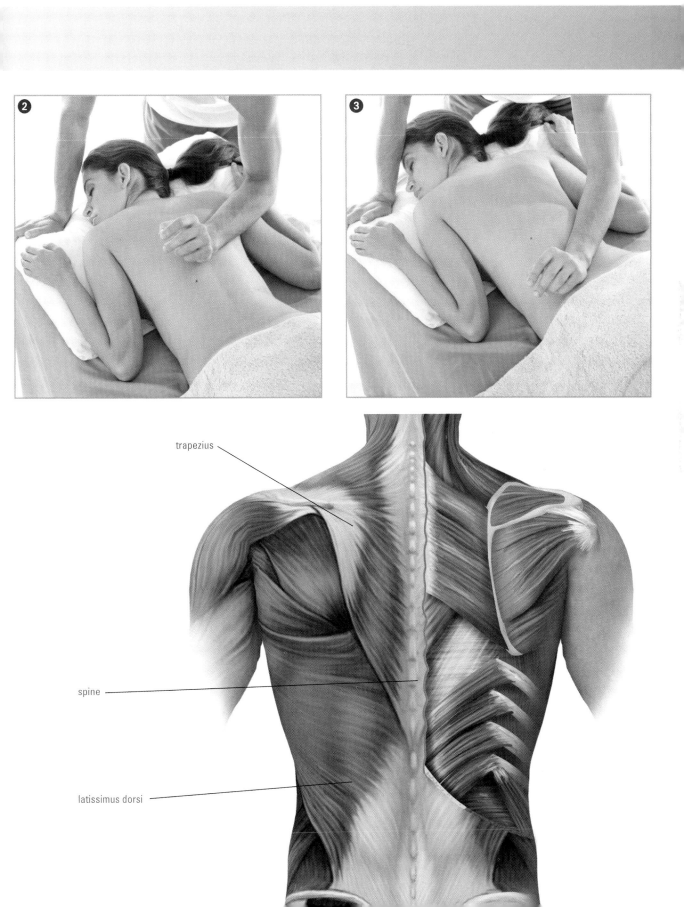

trapezius

spine

latissimus dorsi

THE BACK (CONTINUED)

For the next two massage strokes you'll need to position yourself at your subject's side. Reach over her back and place your hands, one atop the other, on her side.

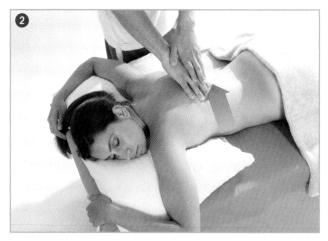

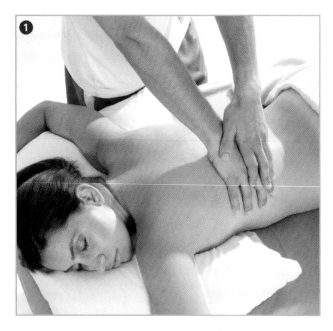

1–2 For the first stroke, firmly but gently pull your flat hand up her side toward her spine. Repeat this a few times on each side of her body. Next, make a "claw" shape with the bottom hand, place your fingertips between her ribs, and pull upward gently but firmly. This move is called "raking the ribs." Repeat several times on each side of her body.

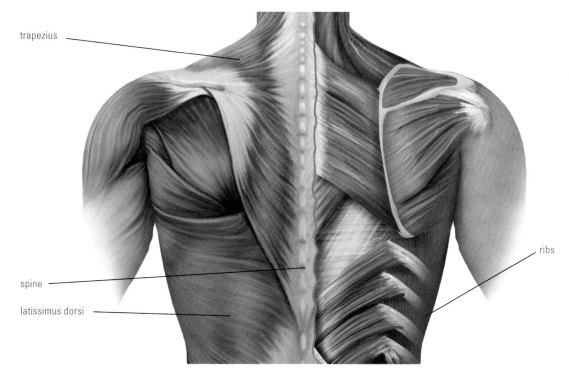

trapezius

ribs

spine

latissimus dorsi

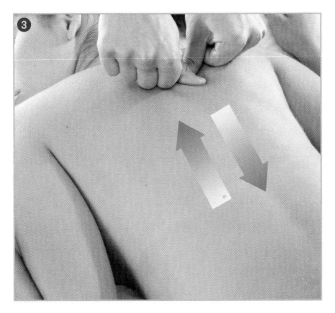

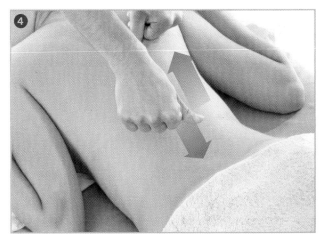

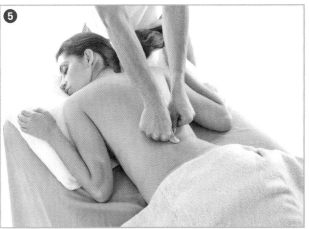

3–**5** While standing in front of one of your subject's shoulders, place your thumbs to one side of her spine. Using firm but gentle pressure, run your thumbs up and down her back, across her trapezius (traps) and latissimus dorsi (lats). This movement is called "stripping" the muscle.

You can move your thumbs together, or move one up and the other down. Repeat several times on each side of her back.

SUPPORT THE THUMBS WHEN STRIPPING THE MUSCLE

To avoid straining your thumb, be sure to support it with the rest of your fingers, as shown here.

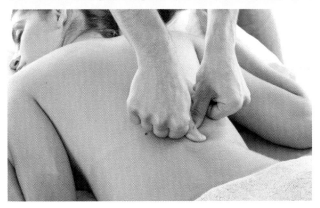

THE BACK (CONTINUED)

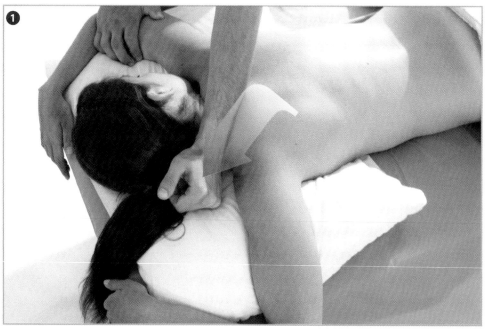

1 Glide the meaty part of your forearm across the back of the shoulder, toward the table. Apply more pressure on the way down than on the way up. Repeat on her other shoulder.

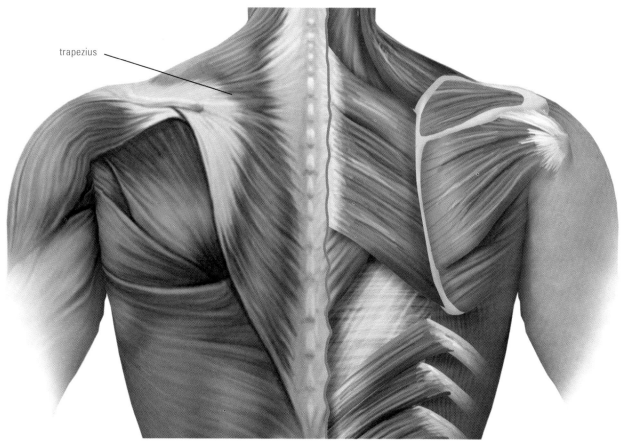

trapezius

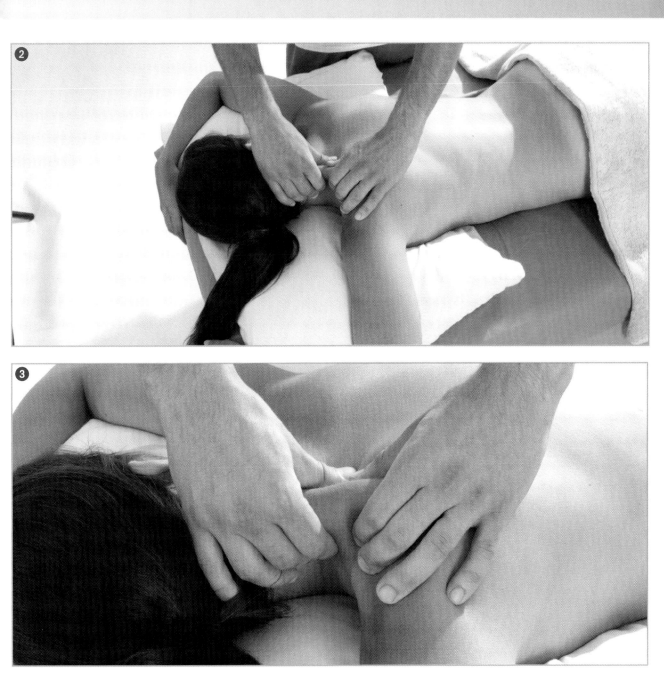

2–**3** Next, squeeze the traps muscle with both hands simultaneously, and then knead the muscle, squeezing first with one hand and then the other, as if you were kneading dough.

THE BACK (CONTINUED)

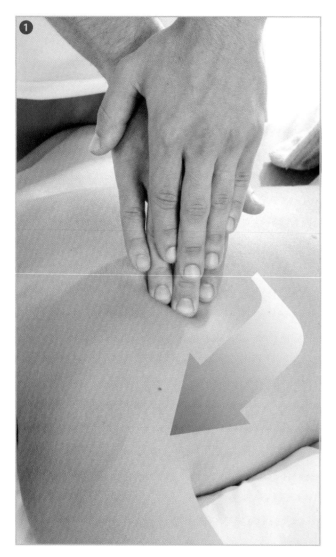

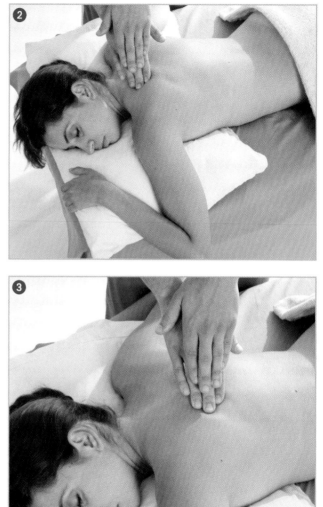

❶–❸ In the next move you'll be pressing your fingertips against the edges of the shoulder blade, or scapula, as you circle it. Place one hand atop the other on the shoulder blade, while gently pressing your fingers in a circular motion around it. This move is called "scraping the scapula."

CAUTION

Always take care—and be very gentle—when massaging around the neck. It's an endangerment zone, with lots of nerves.

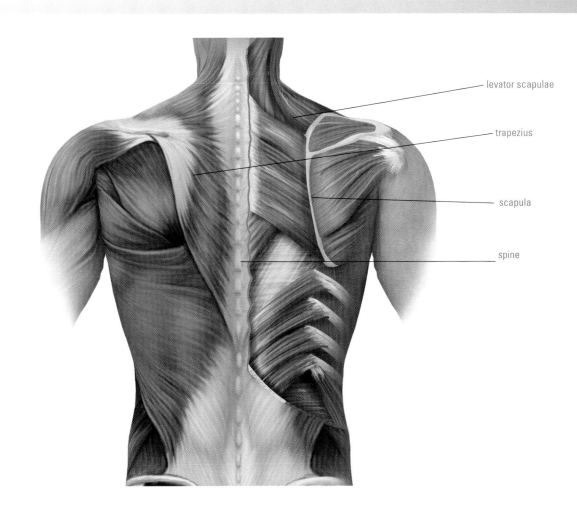

levator scapulae

trapezius

scapula

spine

4 The levator scapulae are the muscles that lift the scapula, or shoulder blade, toward the ears. They're situated at the side and back of the neck, under the trapezius muscles.

Massaging these muscles feels great. That's because almost everyone's levator scapulae are overstretched due to poor posture while sitting and driving and even carrying heavy handbags. To work these muscles, place one hand atop the other and then use firm but gentle pressure to move both back and forth and in circles.

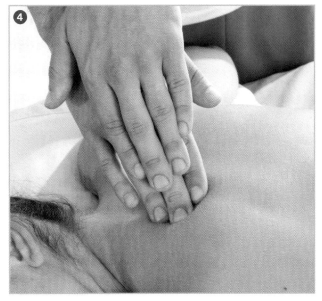

THE BACK (CONTINUED)

1–**3** The spine of the scapula is a plate of bone that runs across the shoulder blade. In this stroke, you'll be working the muscles around that structure.

Place the thumb and fingers of one hand on either side of the spine of the scapula and then run your hand gently along its length. Follow that immediately with the opposite hand, and then the first hand again to continue the motion. Repeat several times on each side.

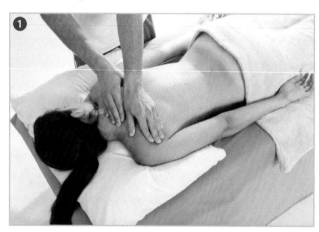

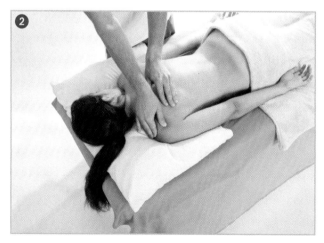

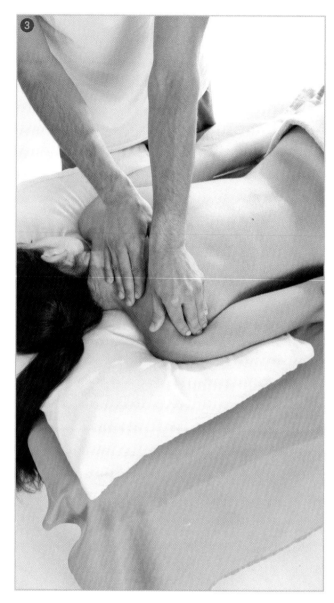

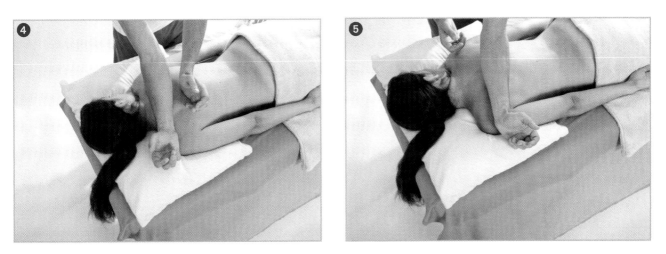

4–**5** Next, run the fleshy part of each forearm along each side of the spine of the scapula, either one and then the other, or both at once.

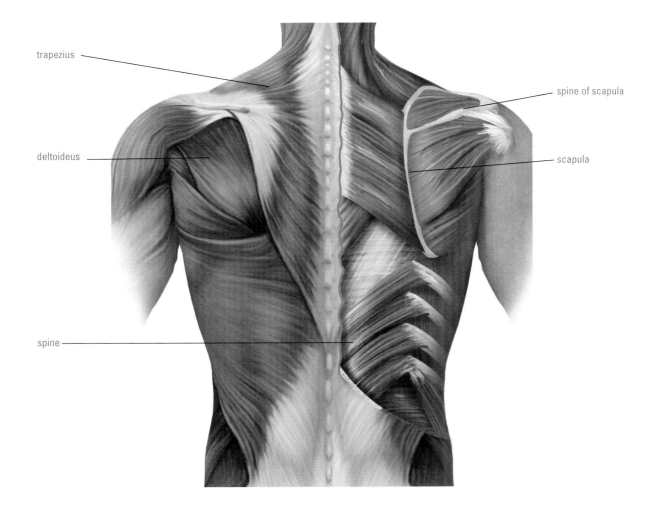

trapezius

deltoideus

spine

spine of scapula

scapula

THE BACK (CONTINUED)

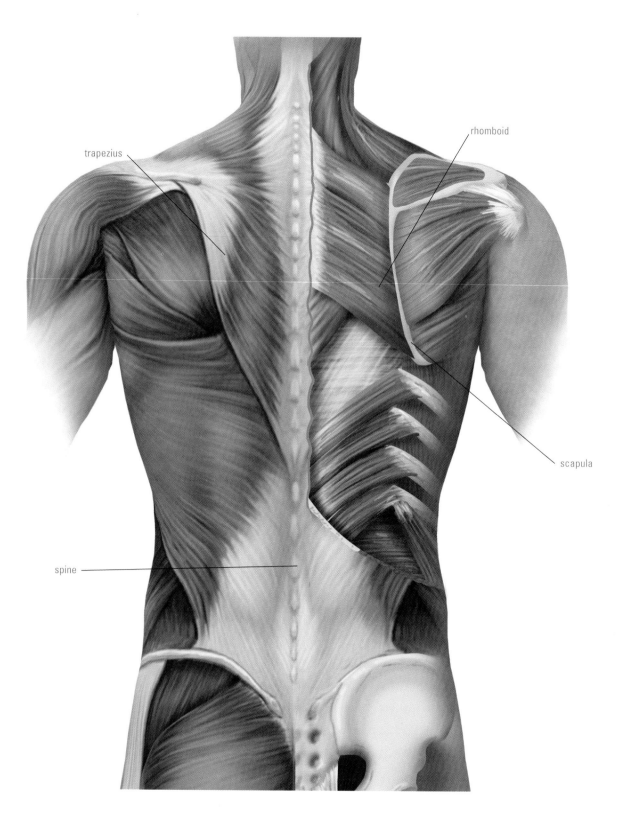

rhomboid

trapezius

scapula

spine

1–**2** For the next move, you'll be working your subject's rhomboid, the muscle under the trapezius that connects the scapula (shoulder blade) to the spinal column. To massage it, place one hand atop the other, press into the muscle (just to the left or right of the spine) with your fingertips, and work back and forth and then in small circles all over the muscle.

CROSS-FIBER FRICTION

Cross-fiber friction, or the technique of working a muscle against its grain, soothes and aligns muscle tissue more quickly than working in line with the grain. Because the rhomboid muscle is typically overstretched in most people, cross-fiber friction can bring relief quickly.

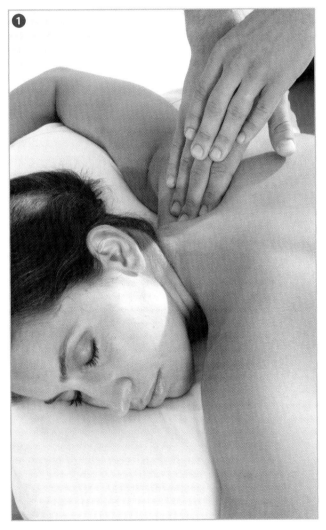

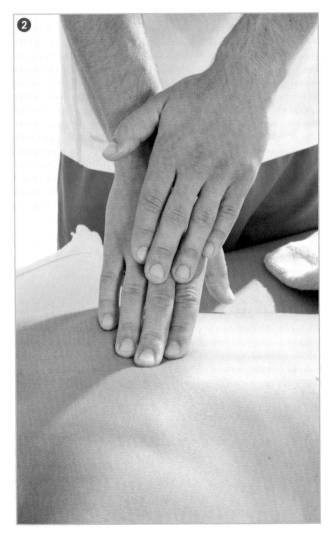

LOWER BACK

In the next few moves you'll be taking the massage to your subject's lower back. Remember that as you move from one body part to another, you want to maintain contact with your subject's body at all times for a smooth and seamless transition.

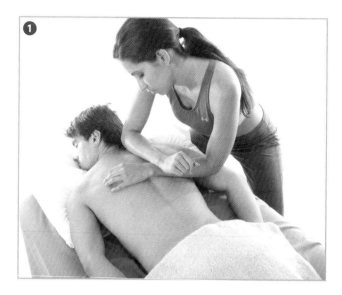

❶–❷ To begin the transition, place your arms on your subject's back as shown, keeping both your wrists relaxed. Make sure both of your arms make contact with your subject's back; this gives your subject the illusion of a "big hand" touching his body. Glide your arms down your subject's back, toward his glutes.

CAUTION

Do not massage the soft area between your subject's last rib and the top of the hip. This is an endangerment zone because the kidneys are located in this area.

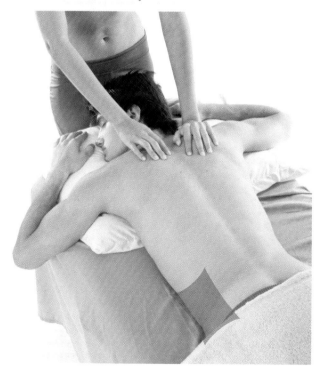

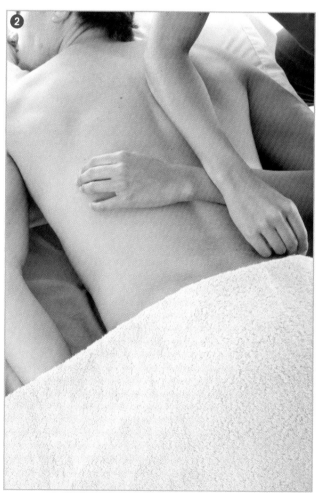

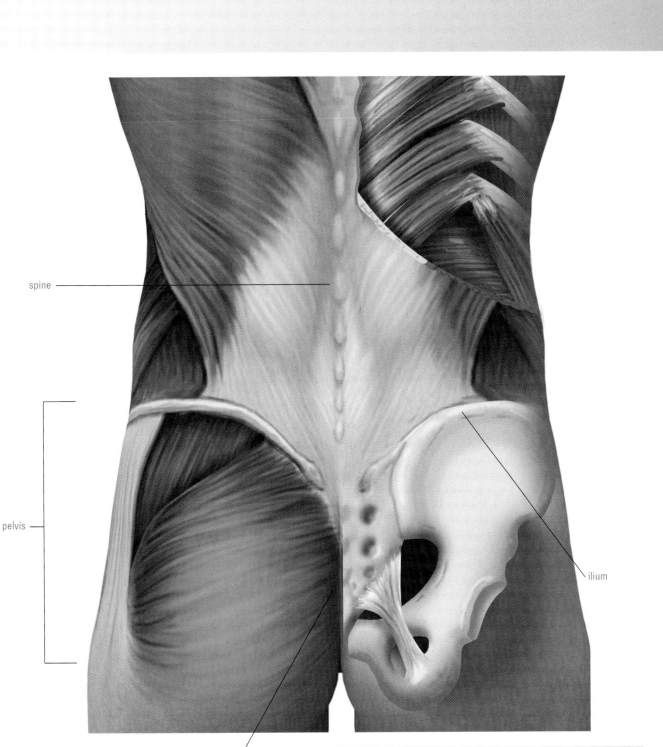

spine

pelvis

ilium

sacrum

PILLOW TALK

During any massage—but especially while his lower back is being worked on—your subject may be more comfortable with a thin pillow under his hips.

LOWER BACK (CONTINUED)

1 The next stroke of the massage is called "scraping the sacrum." The sacrum is the triangular bone at the base of the spine. To do this stroke, place one hand atop the other and press along the sacrum with your fingertips.

In addition to the pressing stroke, you can also rub along the sacrum in a back-and-forth motion or make small circles. After you use your fingertips, you can also use your knuckles or the palms or heels of your hand.

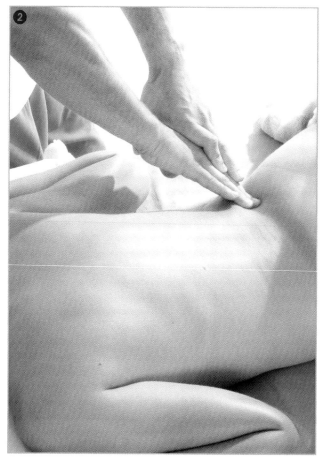

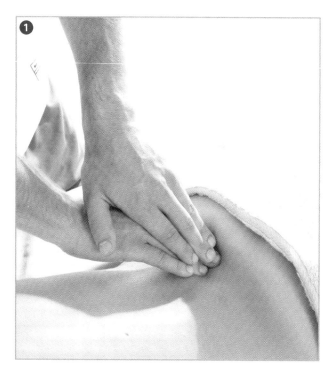

2 Next, use your fingertips as above to "scrape" along the top of the hip bone where it meets the small of the back. Lots of muscles attach in that area. When you work an area at which a muscle attaches, you benefit the entire muscle.

CAUTION

In traditional Chinese medicine, scraping the sacrum pulls energy downward. For that reason, do not do this stroke if your subject is—or even may be—pregnant.

In addition, avoid these sacrum strokes if your subject has sciatica or any disk problems.

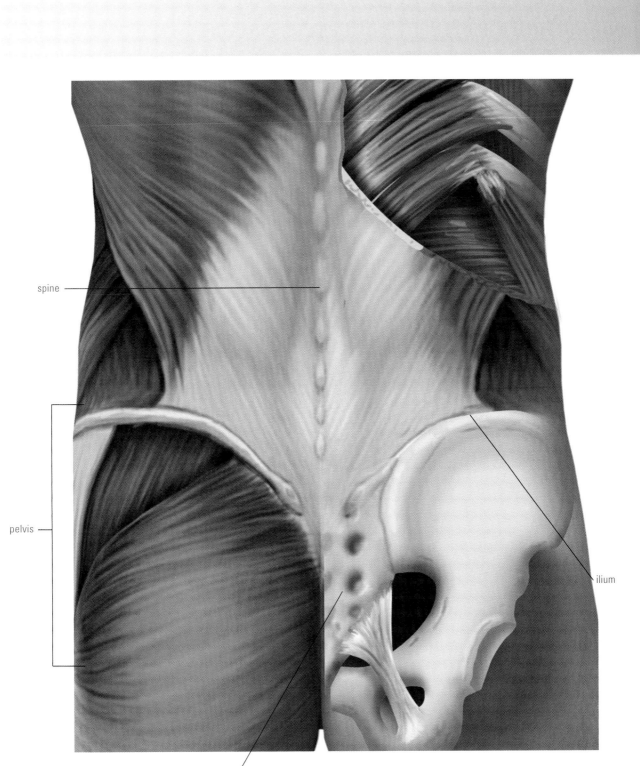

spine

pelvis

ilium

sacrum

②LOWER BODY: BACK

The massage continues over your subject's glutes and legs. Don't be surprised if your subject is ticklish here. If that's the case, our advice is to slow down a bit and use deeper and more deliberate movements. Remember to use care when working the back of the knees.

We close this section with a relaxing foot massage before your subject switches to a face-up position.

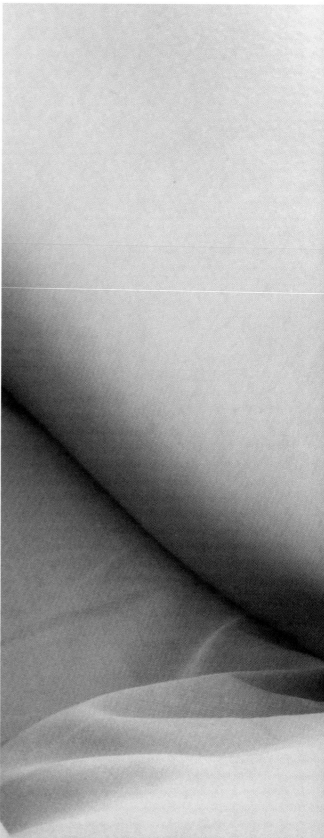

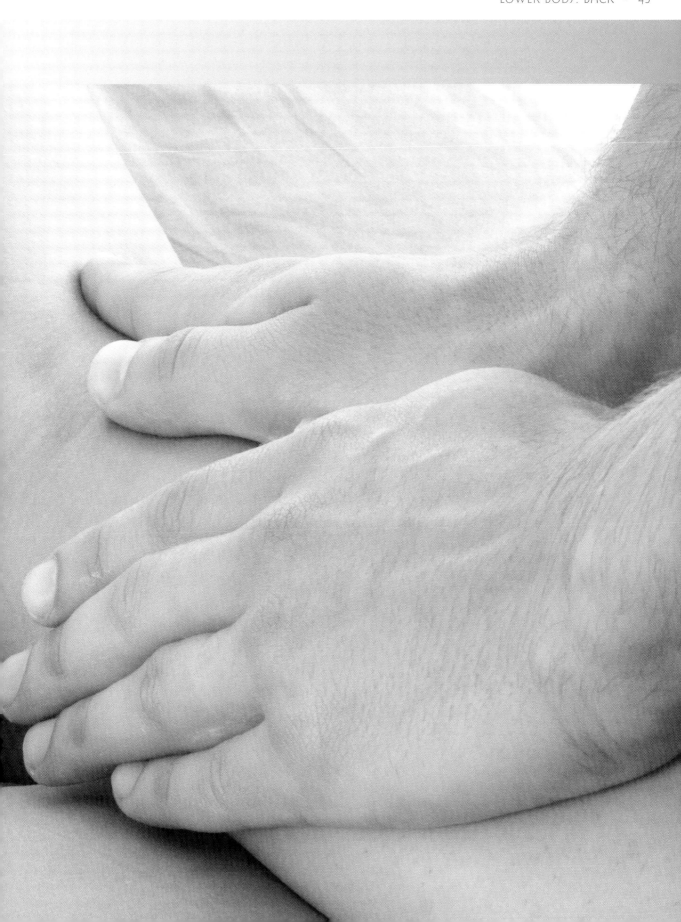

GLUTES

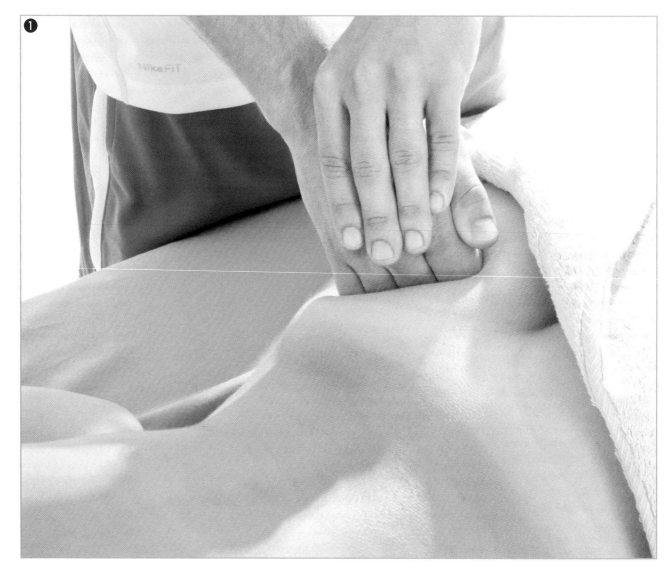

The glutes—also known as your butt muscles—are the largest muscles in your body. Tightness in that area can contribute to discomfort in the lower back. These strokes will help loosen those muscles.

❶ First, make a fist with one hand, and place the first set of knuckles in the space between the top of the greater trochanter and the iliac crest, or hip bone. (This is a good place to work because several muscles attach in that area, and so all of the muscles benefit to some degree.) Support the hand that is making a fist with the other hand, and press the fist into the area.

MASSAGE TIPS

If you feel a bump on a bone, that's where a muscle or tendon is attached. This is usually a good place to work.

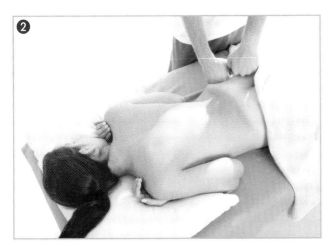

2 Next, make fists with both hands and gently press into the buttocks using a piston motion, pressing with one fist and then the other.

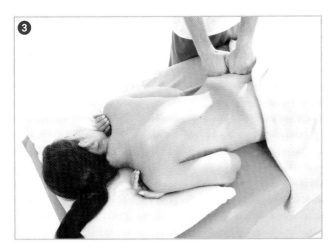

3 To continue, rotate your fists, in the same or opposite direction, into the area. To further work the glute muscles, continue to manipulate the area with your palms and/or fingertips.

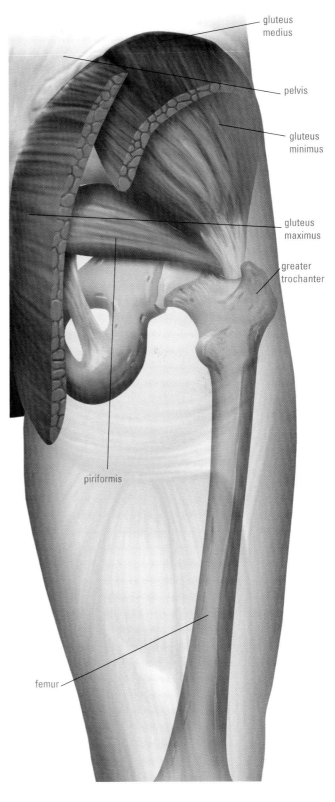

gluteus medius

pelvis

gluteus minimus

gluteus maximus

greater trochanter

piriformis

femur

LEGS

For the next portion of the massage, you'll be moving on to a new part of your subject's body—his or her legs. That means you'll be starting with effleurage again.

Note that you should massage only one leg at a time. In other words, start and finish massaging one leg (and foot) before starting on the other leg.

However, before you pour more oil in your hands, take a minute to drape your subject's back with a sheet to keep her warm.

❶–❺ Now, standing near your subject's feet, warm your hands and the oil. Starting at the ankles, use long strokes up the legs to warm them. Start gently and then gradually increase the amount of pressure you apply.

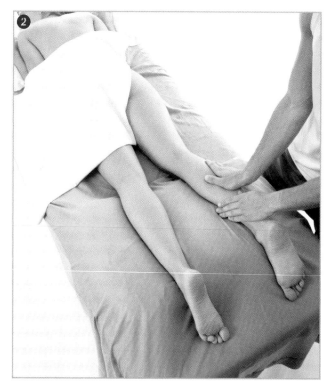

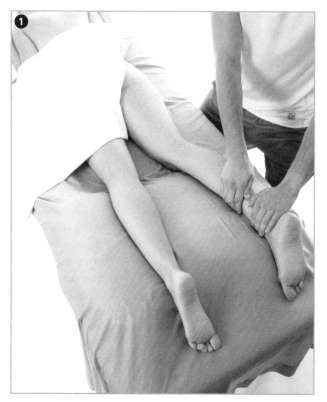

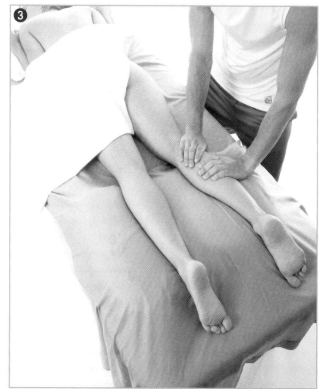

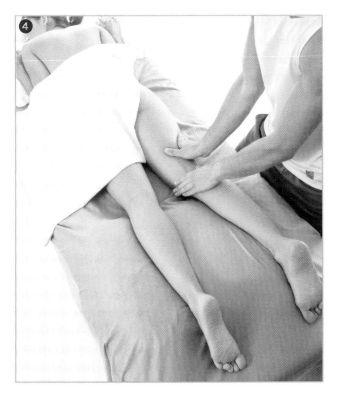

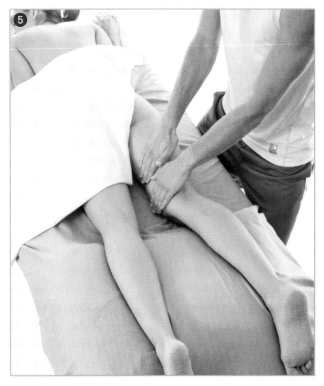

6 When you reach the upper thigh, be sure to work around the greater trochanter, as you did when working the glutes.

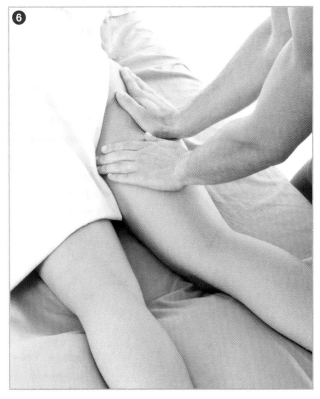

CAUTION

- The inside of the upper leg is an endangerment zone; there are many nerves and blood vessels in the area, so use very light pressure when massaging there.
- The back of the knee is also an area where care needs to be taken. You needn't avoid the area, but you do need to be gentle and apply only very light pressure.
- Do not massage your subject's legs if he or she has varicose veins.
- Do not massage your subject's legs if he or she has recently taken a long plane trip and is experiencing leg pain. This is a symptom of deep-vein thrombosis.

LEGS (CONTINUED)

①–③ Next, place both hands on one of your subject's ankles. Rub your hands back and forth, as if you're wringing a towel—rubbing one hand toward you on the leg as the other hand rubs away from you. Start at your subject's ankles and then work your way up her leg.

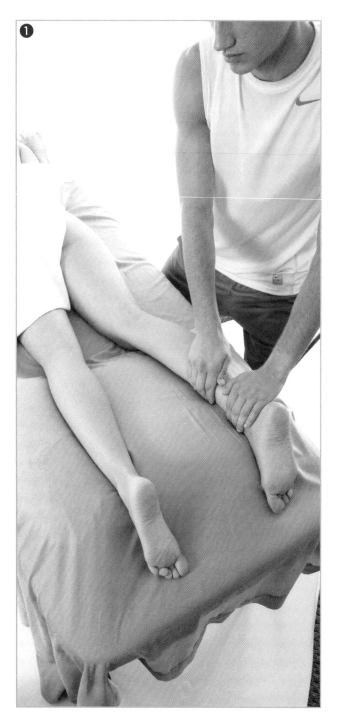

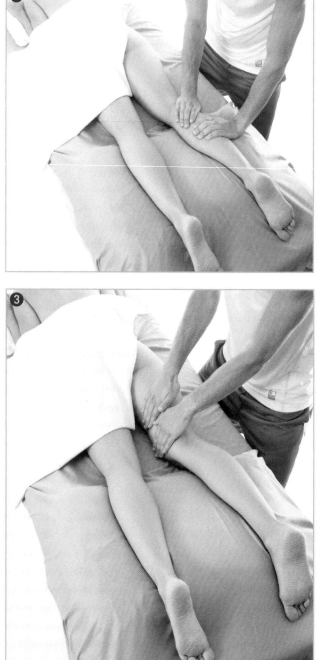

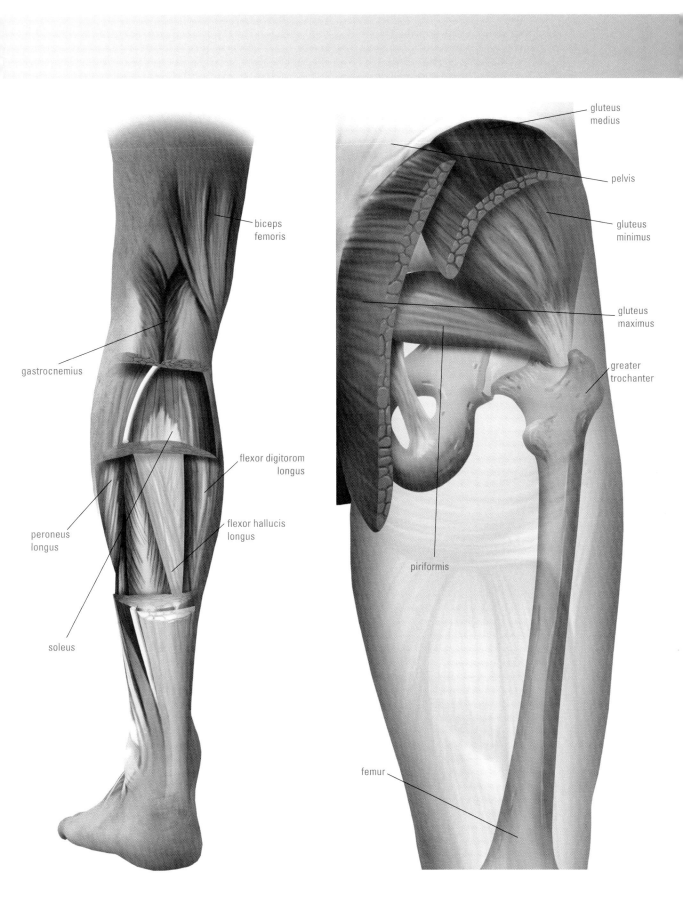

biceps
femoris

gastrocnemius

flexor digitorom
longus

peroneus
longus

flexor hallucis
longus

soleus

gluteus
medius

pelvis

gluteus
minimus

gluteus
maximus

greater
trochanter

piriformis

femur

LEGS (CONTINUED)

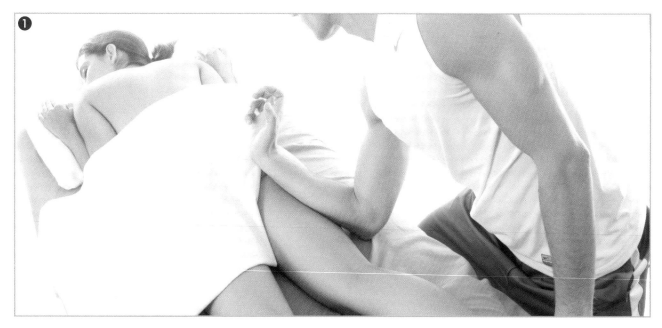

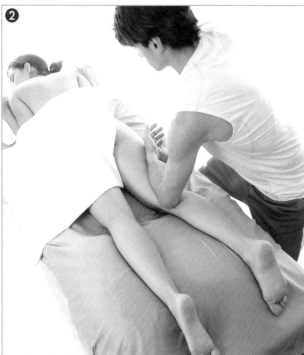

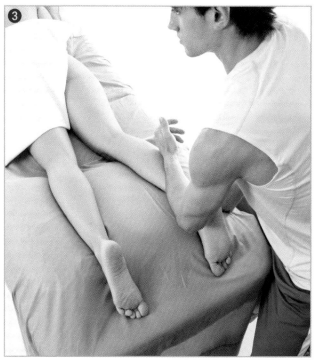

❶–❸ Next, use the meaty part of your forearm to press into the muscles of your subject's leg. This technique works best on the thigh, but you can also work the calves this way as long as you use gentle pressure. When you do, work both the outer calf and the inner calf.

④ Again, when you reach the upper leg, use your forearm to work the muscles in the region around the greater trochanter.

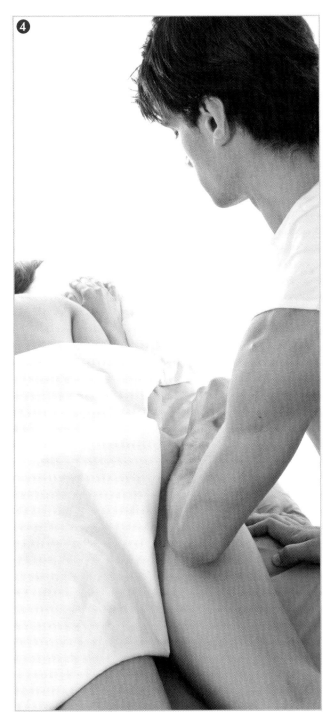

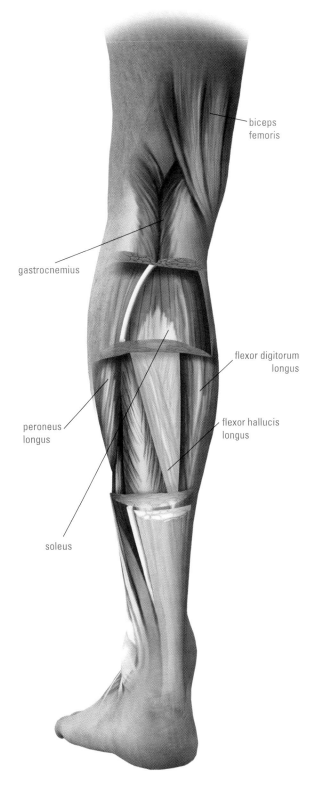

biceps femoris

gastrocnemius

flexor digitorum longus

peroneus longus

flexor hallucis longus

soleus

LEGS (CONTINUED)

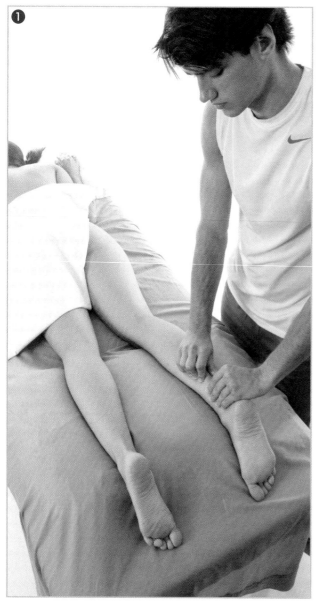

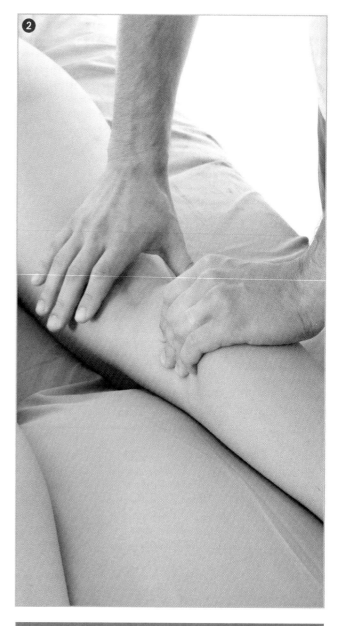

①–**②** Now, knead the leg with both hands—as if you were kneading bread dough—from the ankle to the upper thigh. Squeeze first with both hands simultaneously and then as you squeeze with one hand, release with the other.

TICKLISH?

If your subject is ticklish, work more slowly and deeply.

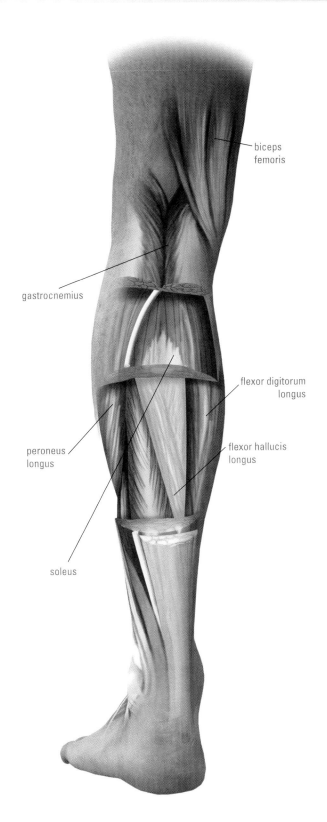

biceps femoris

gastrocnemius

flexor digitorum longus

peroneus longus

flexor hallucis longus

soleus

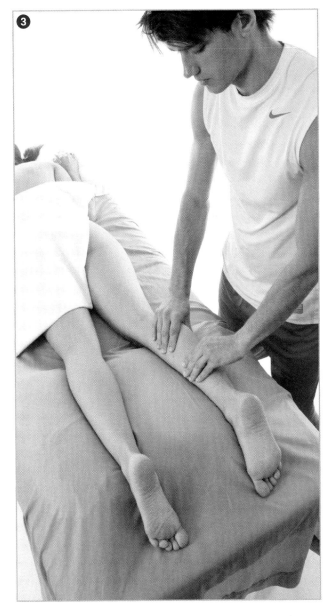

3 Make sure to work very gently at the back of the knee, and don't press too hard.

LEGS (CONTINUED)

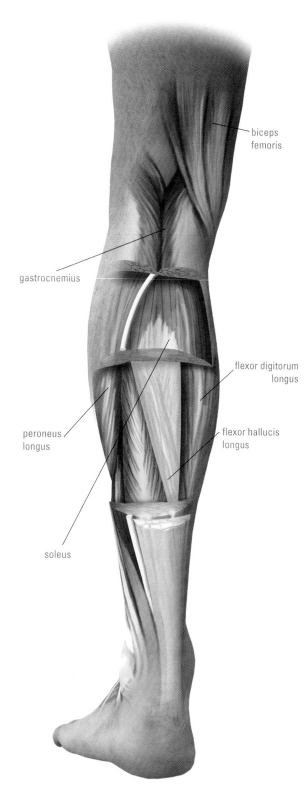

biceps femoris

gastrocnemius

flexor digitorum longus

peroneus longus

flexor hallucis longus

soleus

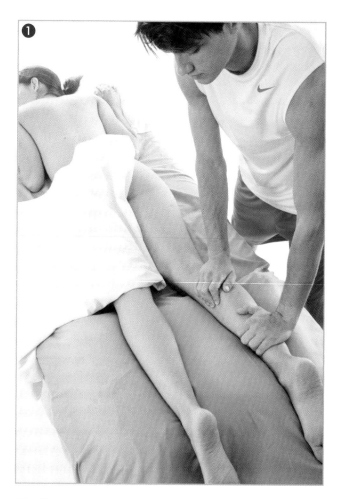

①–③ Next, simply press down on the legs with both hands, beginning at the ankles and working your way up to the upper thigh. Again, take care at the back of the knee, and do not jam your wrists or shoulders.

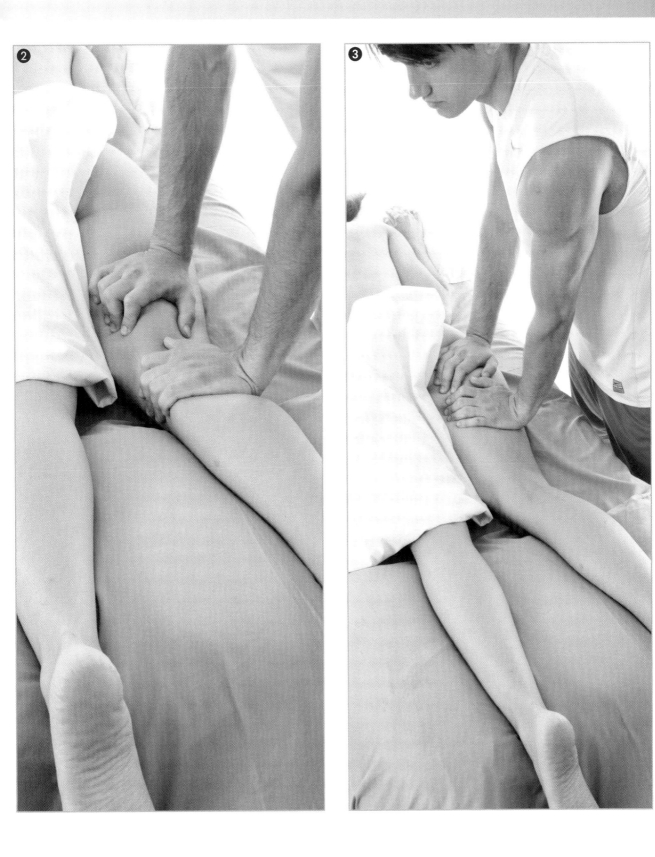

FEET

Most people really enjoy having their feet massaged. That's no surprise, because a good foot massage feels great; so good, in fact, that your whole session could begin and end there.

Entire books have been written about the subject of massaging the feet. (The alternative medical field of reflexology is based on the belief that areas on the foot correspond to areas of the body, and that manipulating areas of the feet can have beneficial health effects.) And hour-long foot massages are not uncommon in the spa world.

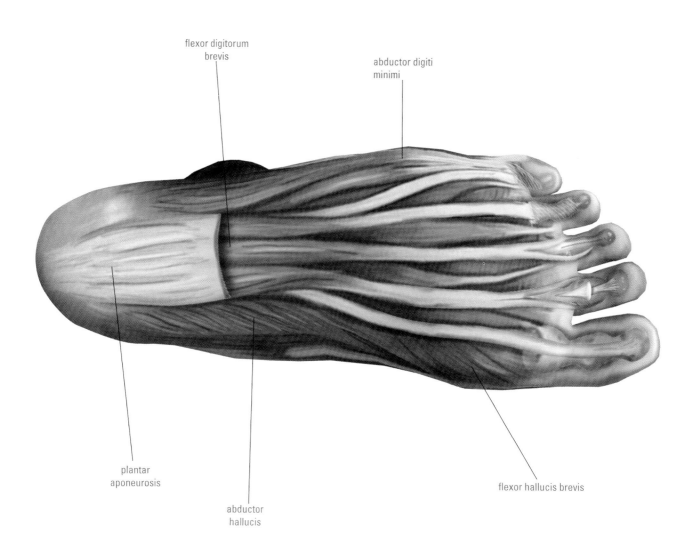

flexor digitorum brevis

abductor digiti minimi

plantar aponeurosis

abductor hallucis

flexor hallucis brevis

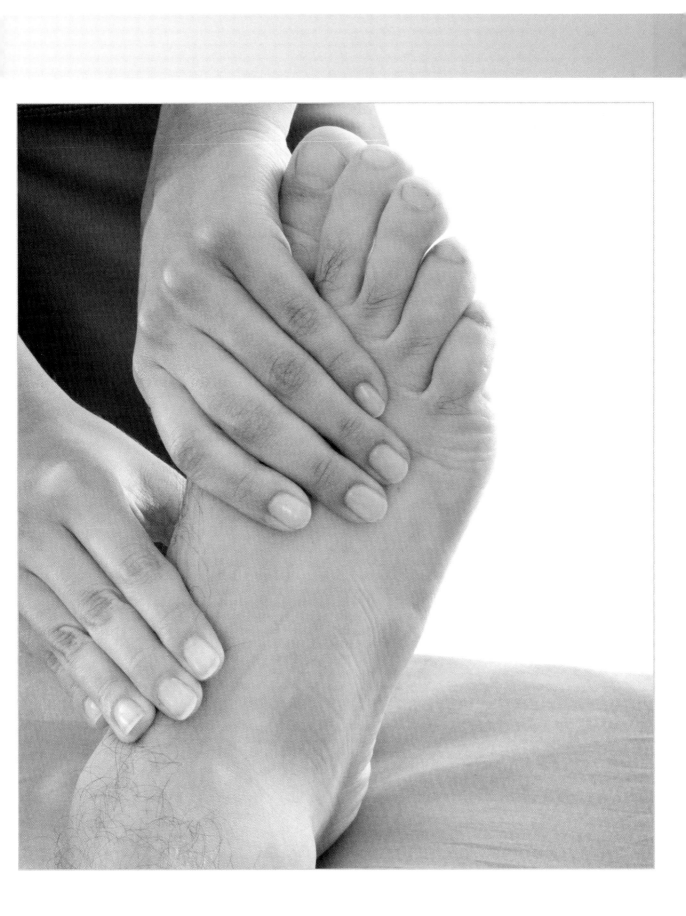

FEET (CONTINUED)

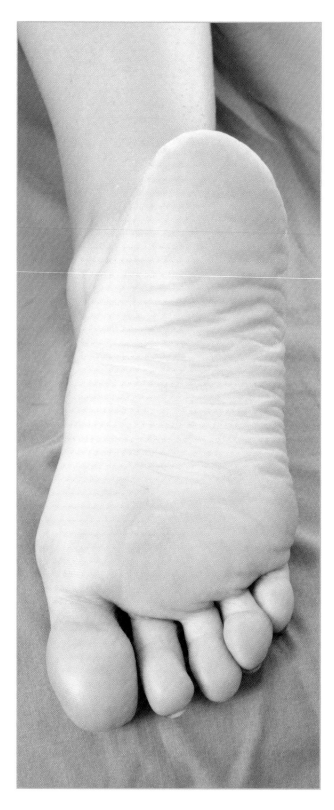

Before you begin, make sure your hands and your subject's feet are clean. (You may want to skip this portion of the massage if your subject has athlete's foot or another fungus, because it's easy to spread it to other parts of his or her body—or even to end up with it yourself.)

If you subject has arthritis, bunions, corns, or calluses, or if his or her toes are misshapen for any reason, be very gentle and careful. Avoid handling ingrown toenails, as they can be quite painful.

If your subject's feet are ticklish, slow down and massage more deeply; that usually eliminates the problem.

Finally, if you're not comfortable massaging feet for any reason, just give your subject's a few squeezes through the sheet and move on to the next body part.

CAUTION

Avoid massaging your subject's foot if she's suffering from an injury or condition such as plantar fasciitis or bone spurs. Unless performed by a qualified physical or massage therapist, working the fascia and muscles of the feet can actually exacerbate injuries. When in doubt, leave it to the pros.

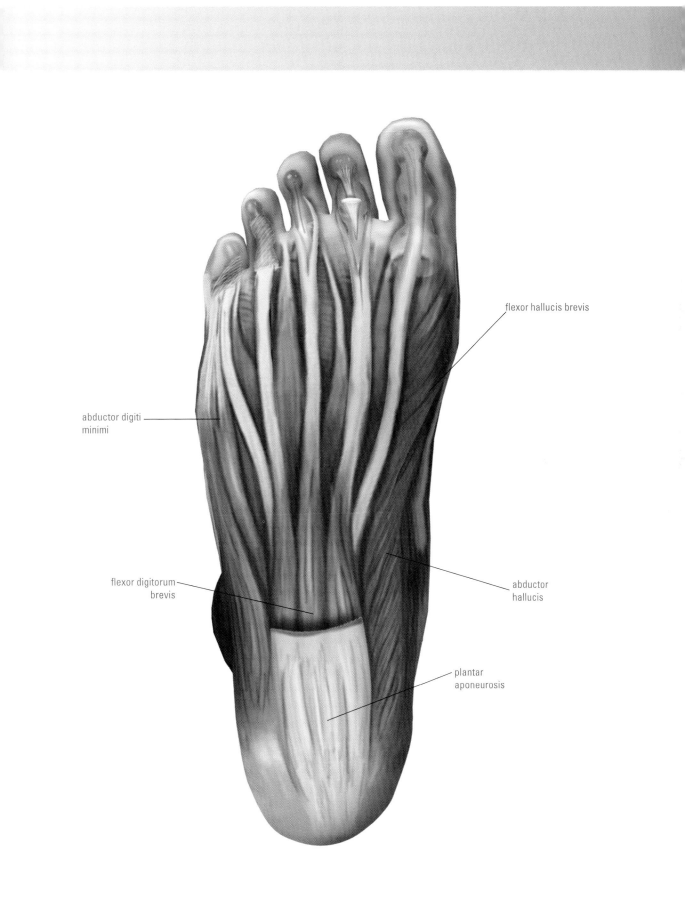

flexor hallucis brevis

abductor digiti
minimi

flexor digitorum
brevis

abductor
hallucis

plantar
aponeurosis

FEET (CONTINUED)

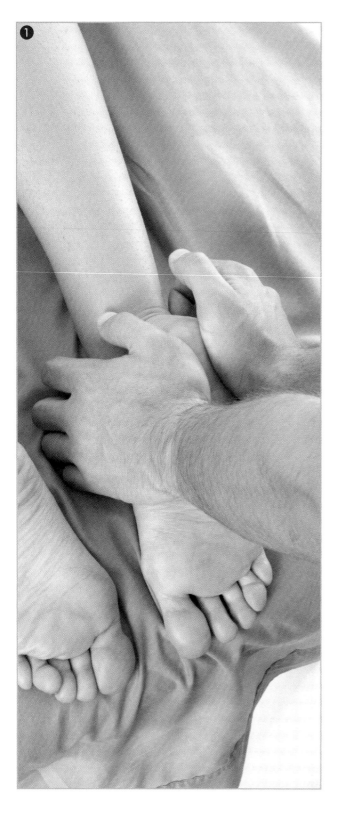

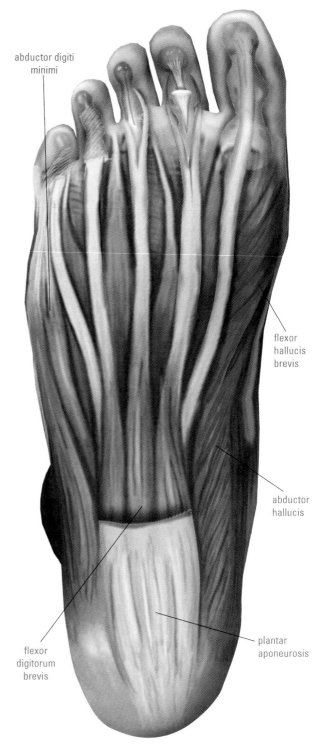

abductor digiti minimi

flexor hallucis brevis

abductor hallucis

flexor digitorum brevis

plantar aponeurosis

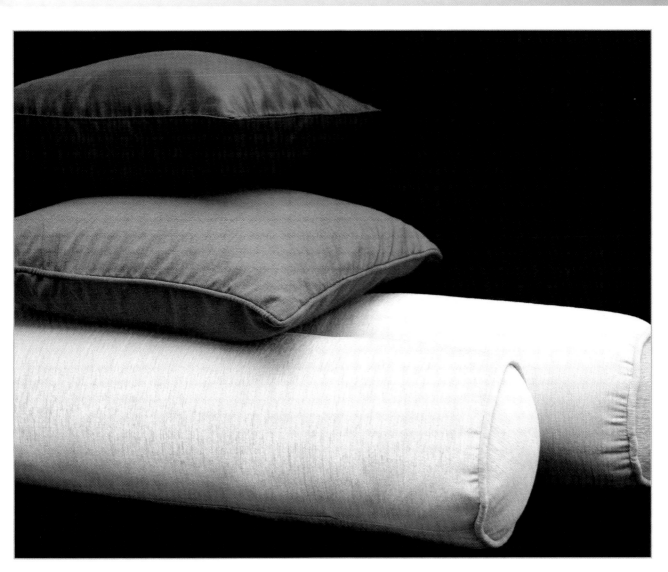

If you haven't already placed a bolster under your subject's ankles, do so before you start the foot massage.

❶ Warm some oil between your hands and then start by pulling one of your subject's feet, hand over hand as if you were pulling a rope.

FEET (CONTINUED)

❶–❷ Next, make a soft fist, and then rub the flat part of your knuckles along the bottom of each foot. As long as your subject's ankles are supported by the bolster, you can use fairly firm pressure. (Ask your subject to let you know if you're using too much.)

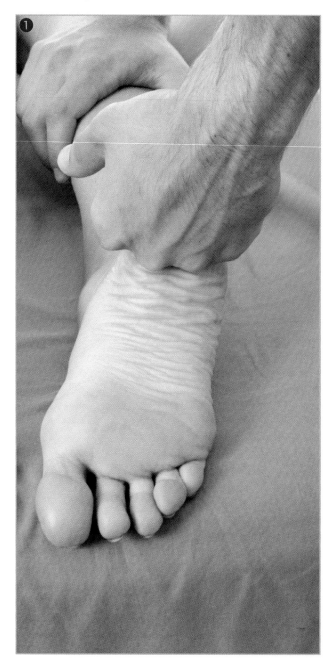

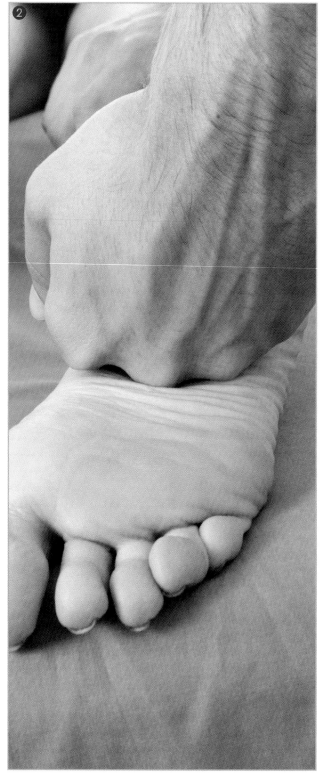

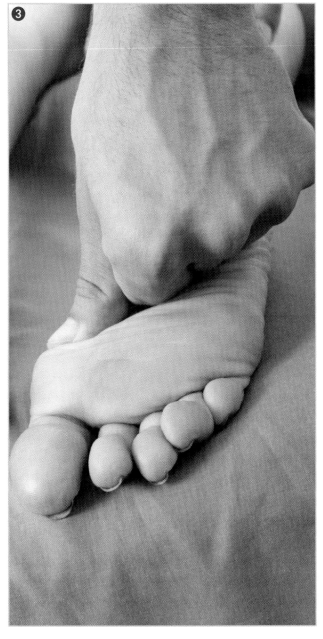

3 Now, run your thumb along the bottom of the foot, from the heel to the end of each of your subject's toes. (Make sure to support your thumb with the rest of your hand). When you reach the end of each toe, press down on its padding; it feels really good.

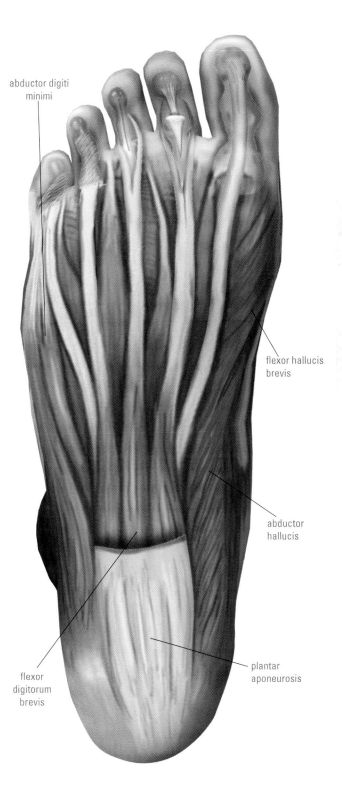

abductor digiti minimi

flexor hallucis brevis

abductor hallucis

plantar aponeurosis

flexor digitorum brevis

FEET (CONTINUED)

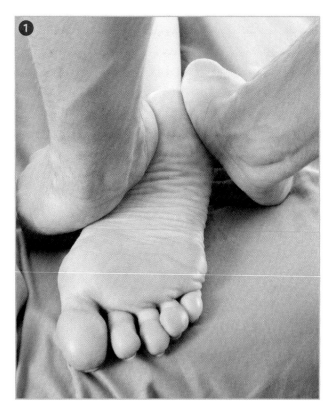

1 Place one hand on each side of one of your subject's feet and rub vigorously back and forth. You're not pulling the foot; rather, you're rubbing the foot between your hands, as if you were trying to warm it up. Start at your subject's ankles and work your way down to the toes.

2 Now hold one of your subject's feet at the arch. Use your other hand to pulse-squeeze each toe.

Next, have your subject switch to a face-up position.

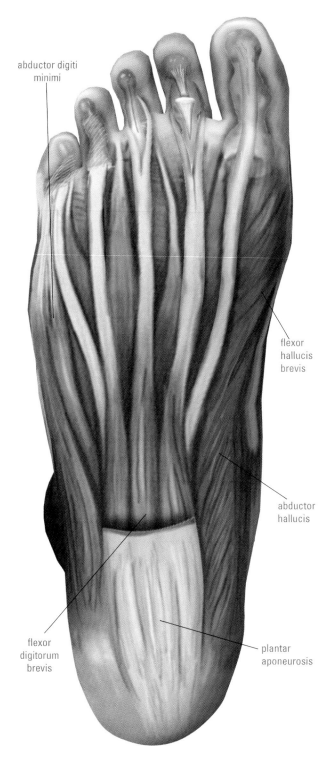

abductor digiti minimi

flexor hallucis brevis

abductor hallucis

flexor digitorum brevis

plantar aponeurosis

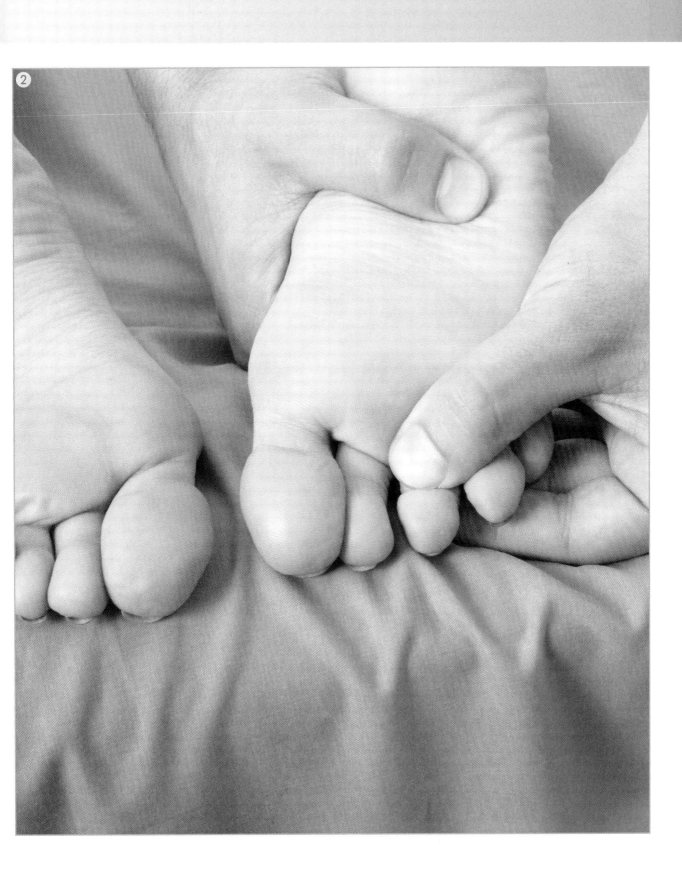

③ LOWER BODY: FRONT

After a long day of exercise, travel, or work, the lower body is often the most easily fatigued. We depend on our legs, knees, and feet to support us during all activities and carry us wherever we need to go. It's no wonder this part of the body is frequently in need of repair and relief. Be careful, though—you may discover that even the least sensitive people are quite ticklish in delicate areas like the soles of the feet.

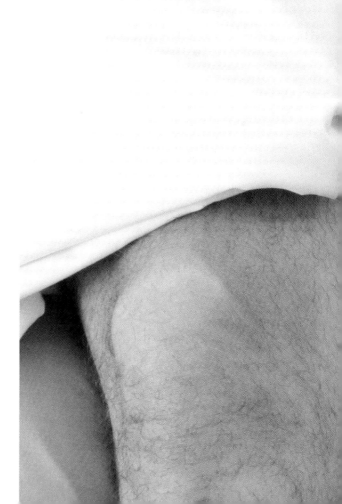

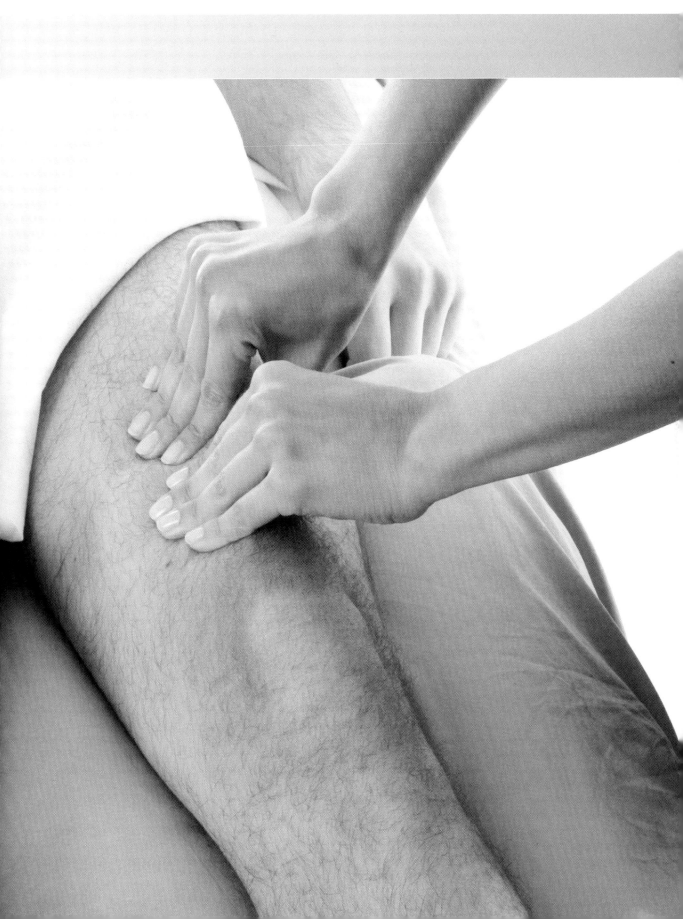

FEET

Before you continue the massage from the face-up position, here are some points to keep in mind.

Some people get a chill when they turn over and lie on their backs, so it's a good idea to have a light blanket nearby.

Your subject can place his arms in any position that is comfortable.

Your subject may want a pillow under his head, but it is not necessary. Likewise, he may like an eye pillow.

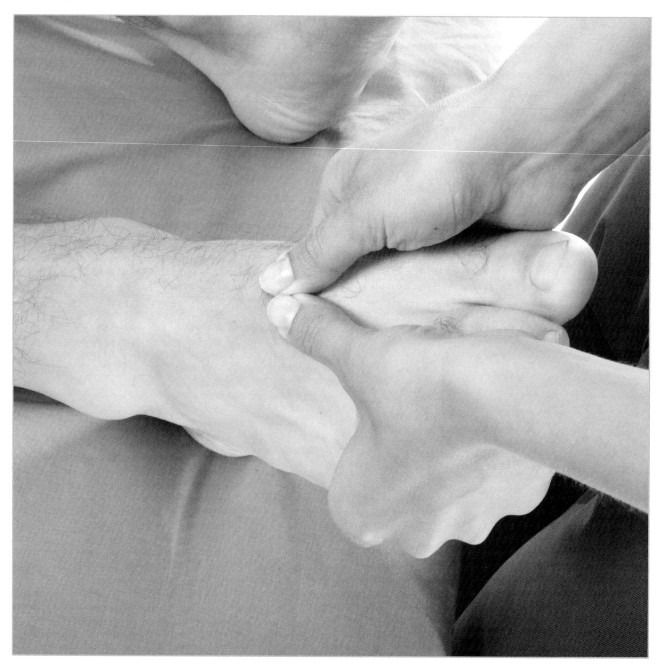

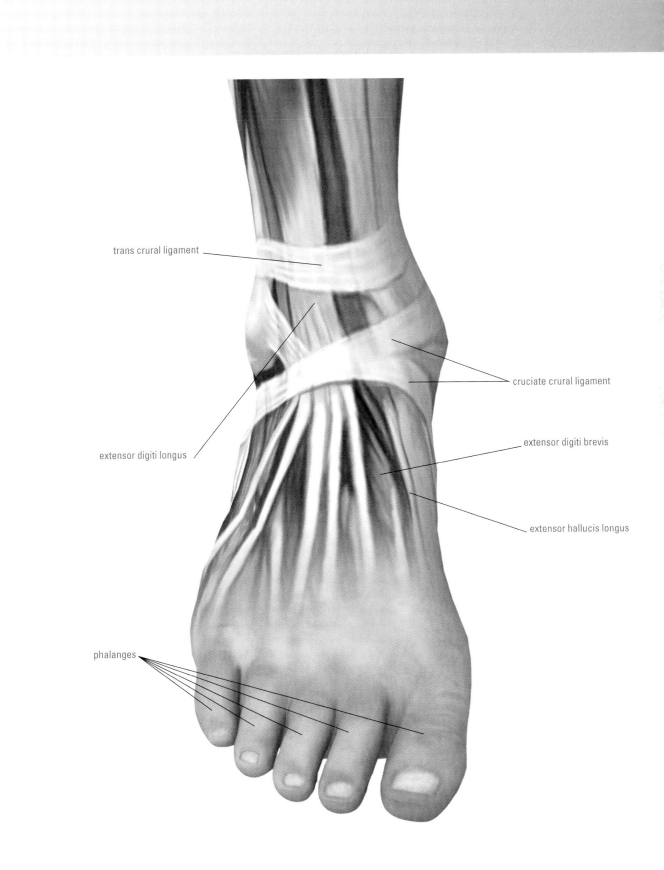

trans crural ligament

cruciate crural ligament

extensor digiti longus

extensor digiti brevis

extensor hallucis longus

phalanges

FEET (CONTINUED)

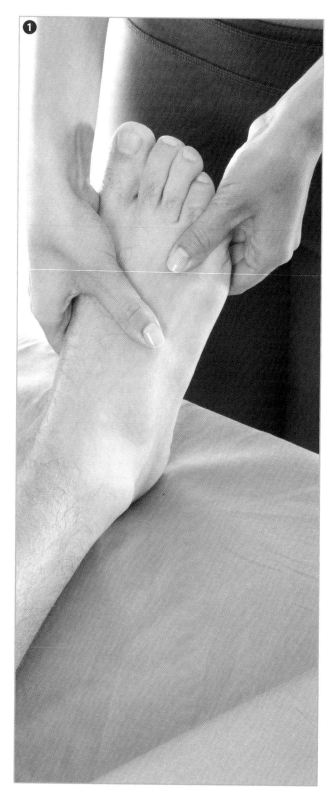

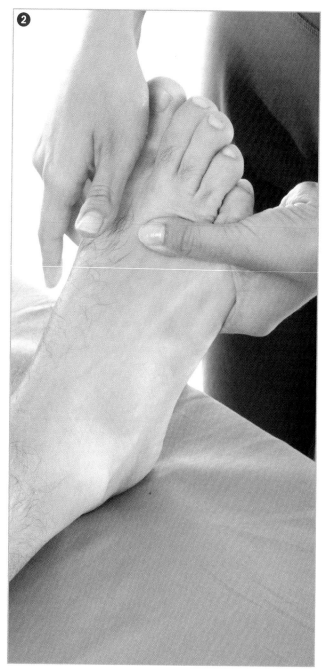

1–3 Once you and your subject are comfortable, continue with the foot massage. Standing at the base of the table, pull on one of your subject's feet, hand over hand, as if you were pulling a rope.

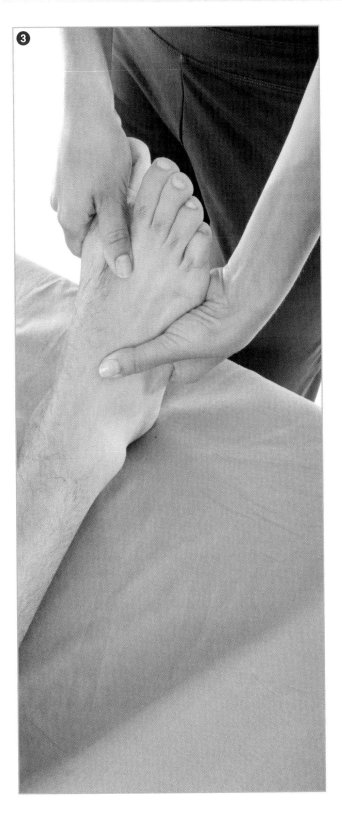

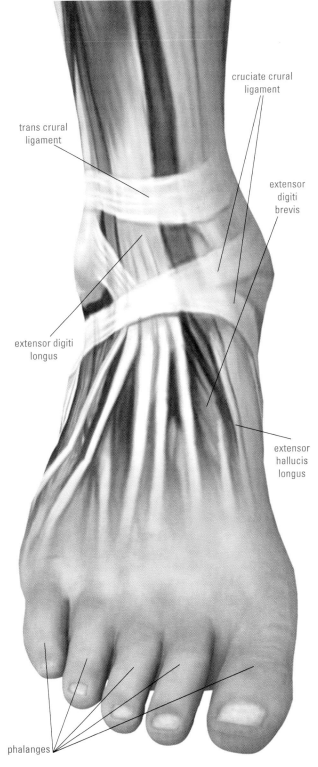

trans crural
ligament

cruciate crural
ligament

extensor
digiti
brevis

extensor digiti
longus

extensor
hallucis
longus

phalanges

FEET (CONTINUED)

1–**3** Next, apply pressure to the sole of each foot with your thumbs. Again, if your subject seems ticklish, go more slowly and apply more pressure.

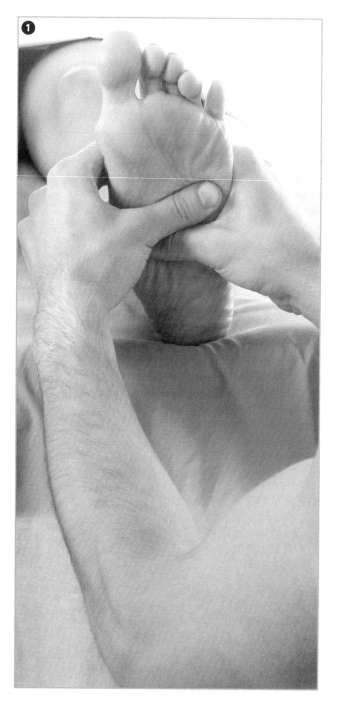

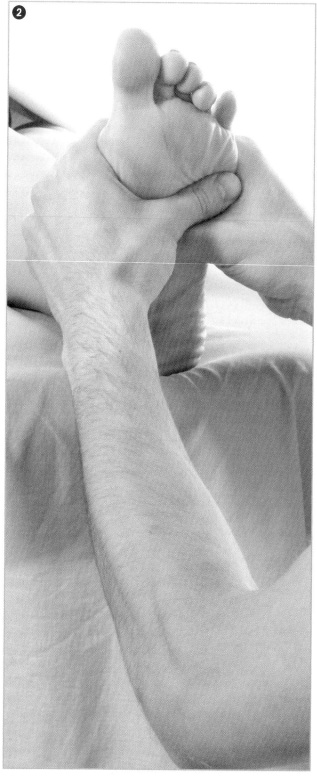

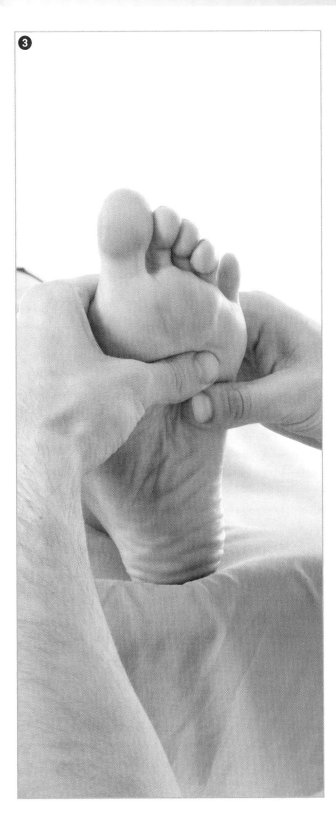

3

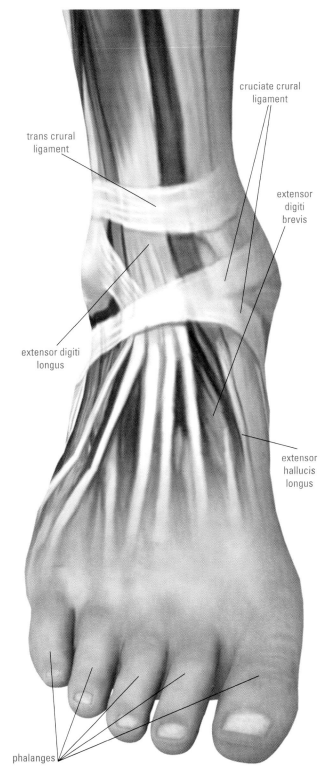

cruciate crural
ligament

trans crural
ligament

extensor
digiti
brevis

extensor digiti
longus

extensor
hallucis
longus

phalanges

FEET (CONTINUED)

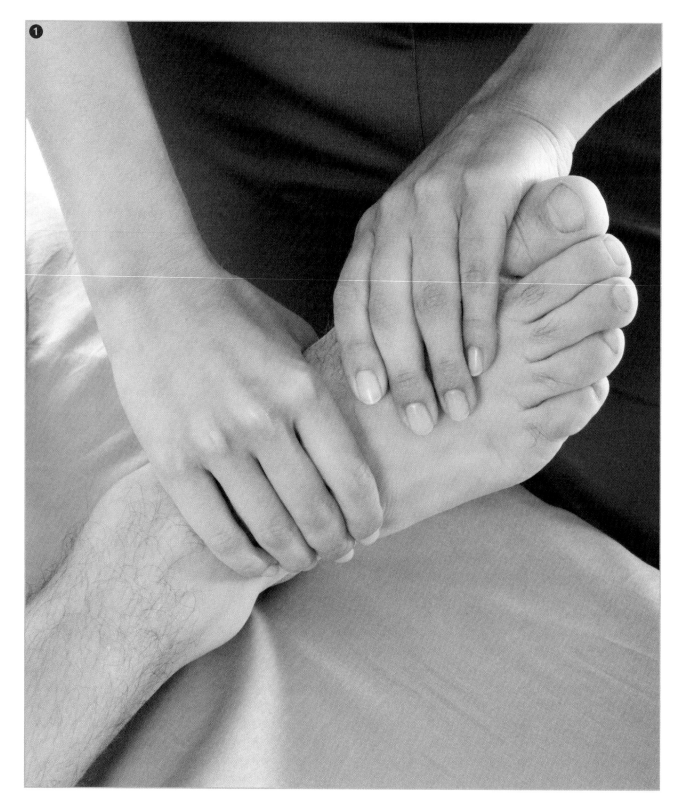

1–**2** This next move requires a little care. Hold your subject's foot near the arch. Now gently "wring" the foot by rotating your hands in opposite directions, without allowing your hands to glide over the skin.

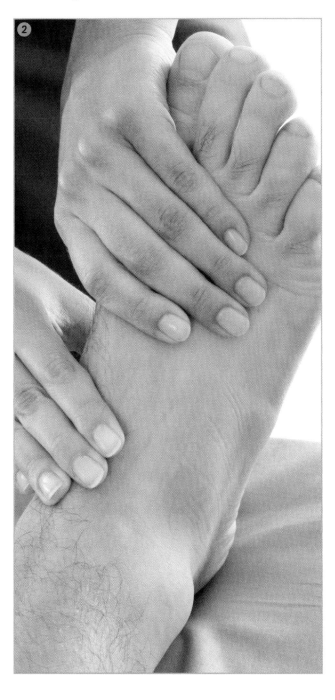

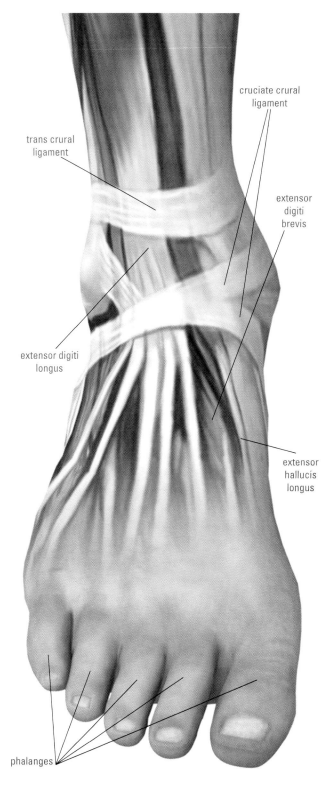

cruciate crural ligament

trans crural ligament

extensor digiti brevis

extensor digiti longus

extensor hallucis longus

phalanges

FEET (CONTINUED)

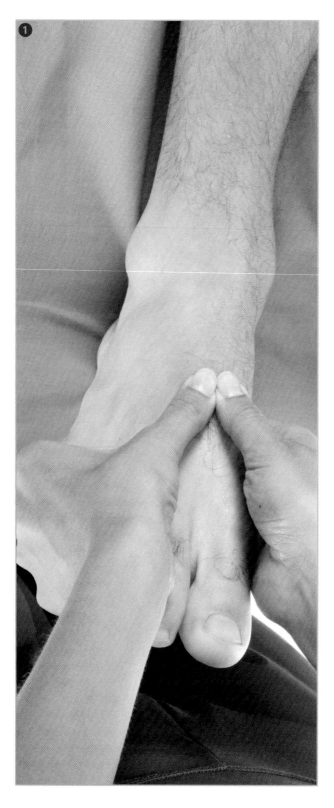

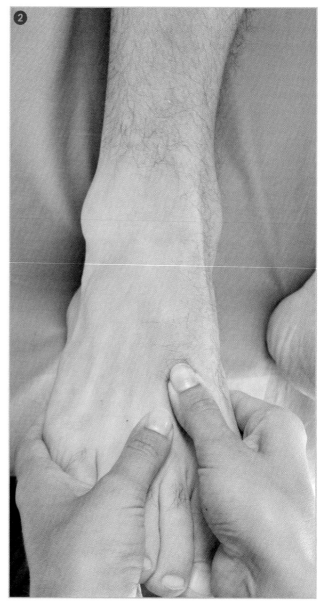

1–**2** Next, you'll "strip" the muscles between the metatarsals—the long bones in the foot. Stand at your subject's feet and grasp one, with your fingers on his arches. Apply pressure with your thumbs between each set of metatarsals and strip the muscles from the ankle to the web between each set of toes. You can work your thumbs in the same or opposite direction.

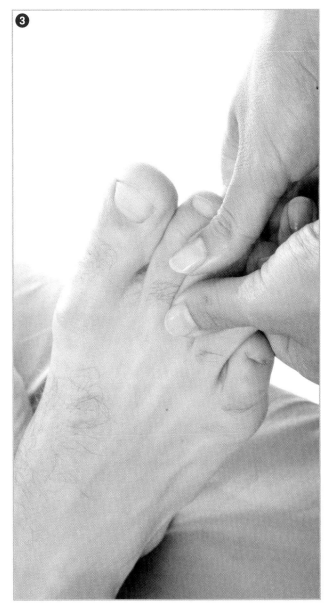

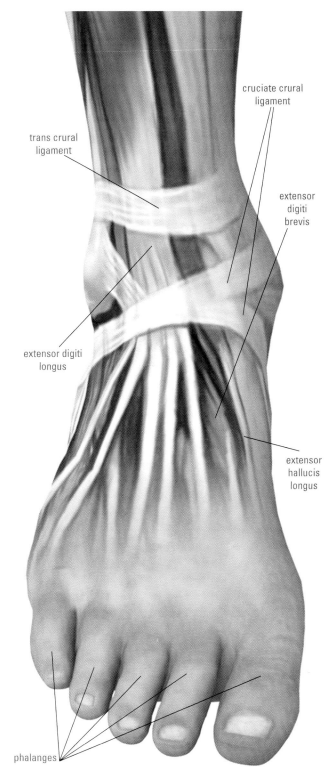

cruciate crural
ligament

trans crural
ligament

extensor
digiti
brevis

extensor digiti
longus

extensor
hallucis
longus

phalanges

3 Now massage each toe with your fingers. You can do this by simply squeezing and pulling each toe or by pulsing the squeezes as you go along the length of each one.

FEET (CONTINUED)

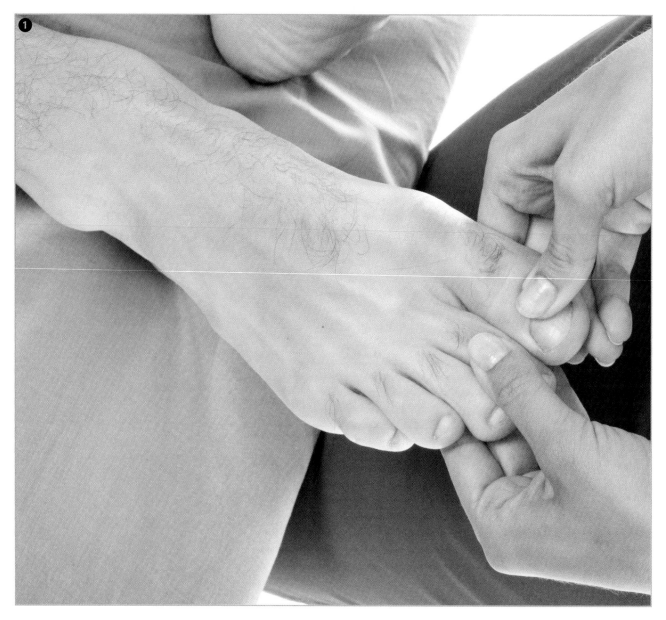

1 Finally, end the foot massage by applying pressure to the base of each toenail.

2 Once you're finished, repeat the entire sequence on your subject's other foot.

CAUTION

If your subject is or may be pregnant, don't do this portion of the massage. The toenails are acupressure points that draw energy down.

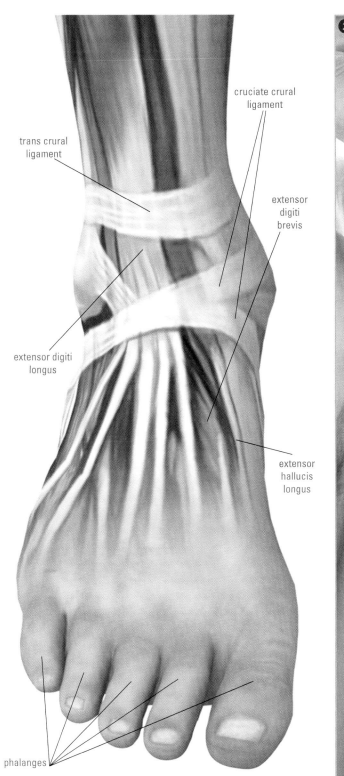

trans crural
ligament

cruciate crural
ligament

extensor
digiti
brevis

extensor digiti
longus

extensor
hallucis
longus

phalanges

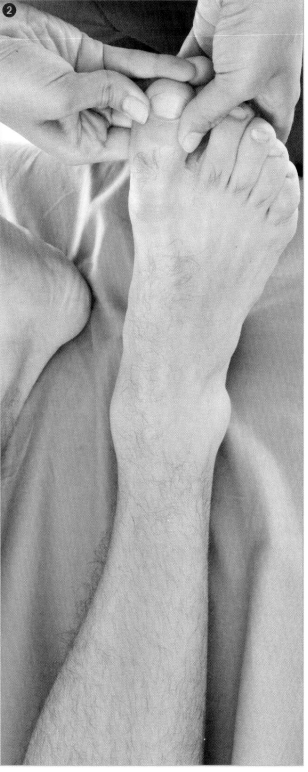

FRONT OF LEGS

Together, the muscles of the legs form one of your body's four largest muscle groups (the others being the muscles of the back, arms, and chest). Without our legs, we wouldn't be able to walk, run, climb, or even sit, and those are reasons enough to treat them well. These massage strokes will help you do just that for your subject.

CAUTION

- During the massage, it's important that you not reach awkwardly, because you could strain your own muscles. Move around to maintain a comfortable posture if you need to.

- Do not massage your subject's legs if he has recently taken a long plane trip and is experiencing leg pain. That could be a symptom of deep-vein thrombosis.

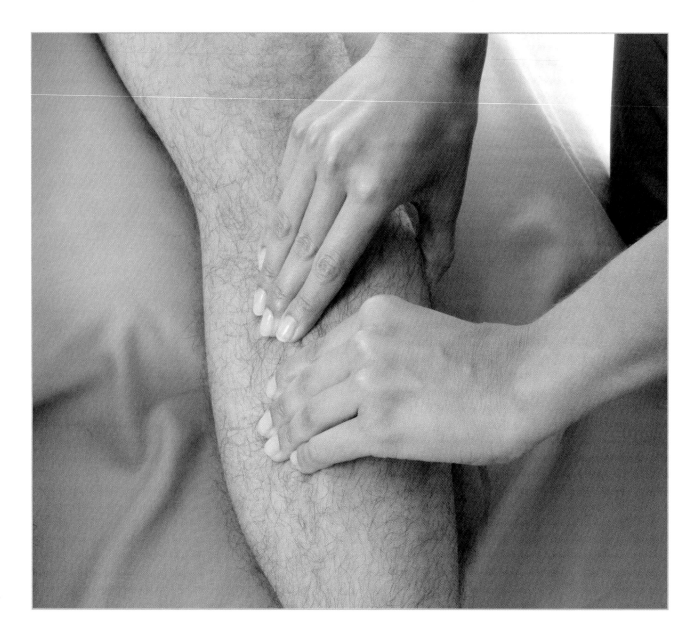

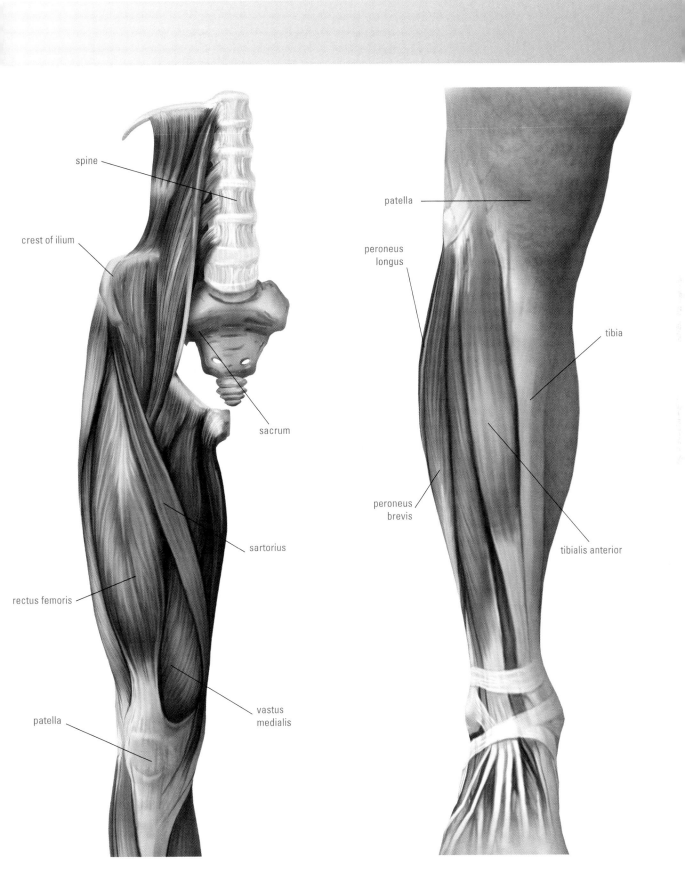

spine

crest of ilium

sacrum

sartorius

rectus femoris

vastus medialis

patella

patella

peroneus longus

peroneus brevis

tibia

tibialis anterior

FRONT OF LEGS (CONTINUED)

①–③ To begin, warm some oil between your hands. Then, standing at your subject's feet, begin with some gentle effleurage strokes to warm the skin and get the blood flowing. Begin very lightly and then gradually increase the amount of pressure you apply.

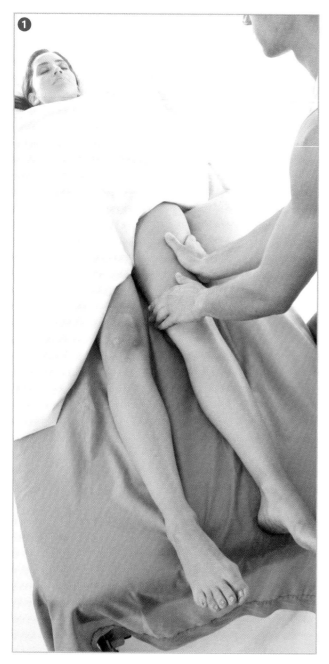

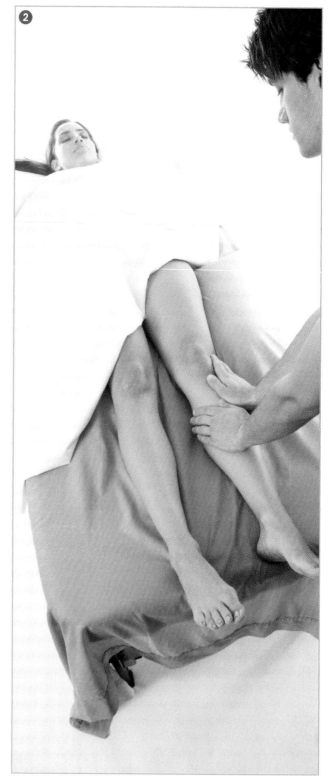

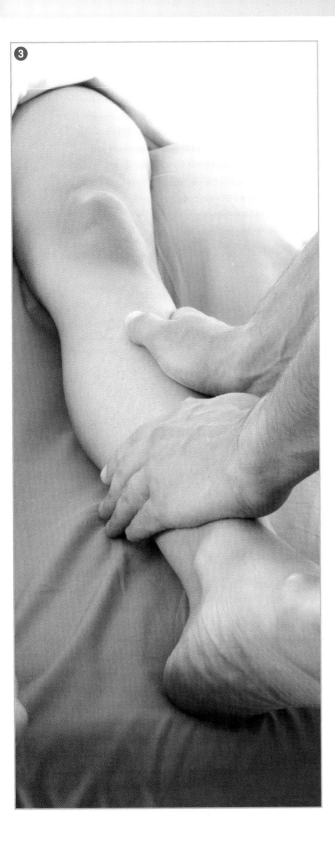

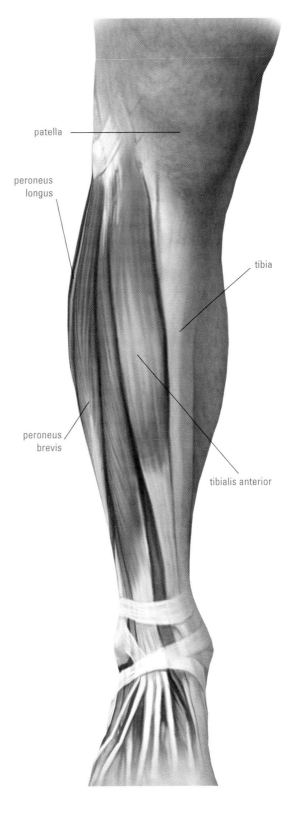

patella

peroneus
longus

tibia

peroneus
brevis

tibialis anterior

FRONT OF LEGS (CONTINUED)

1 Next, squeeze and knead the inside calf muscle, also known as the inner, or medial, gastrocnemius. This is a powerful muscle that works hard, helping us stand, walk, and run—so massaging it feel very good.

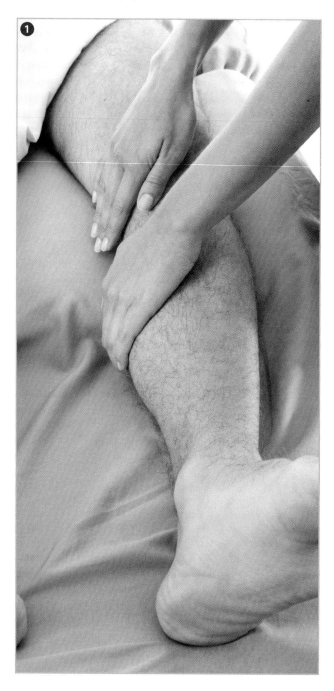

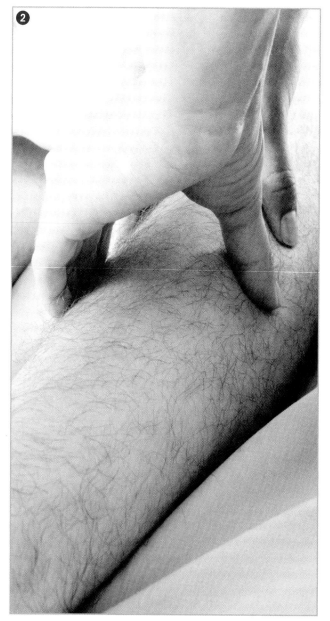

2 Next, use your thumbs to apply friction across the grain of the peroneus longus, the muscle on the outside of the lower leg. Do not do this massage stroke—which relaxes that muscle—if your subject suffers from lots of twisted ankles. Some twisted ankles are caused by an overly loose peroneus longus.

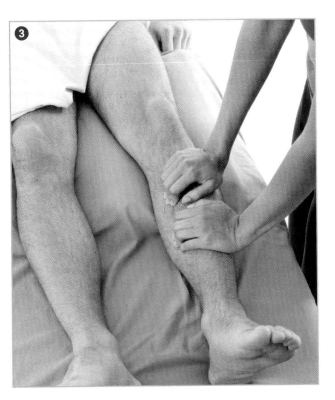

3–**4** Now, gently squeeze along the shinbone, or tibia. Keep in mind that there is not much muscle or fat along that bone, so a light touch is required.

If your subject is suffering from shin splints or has in the past, make sure to massage toward the bone only.

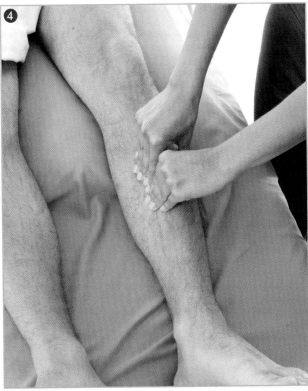

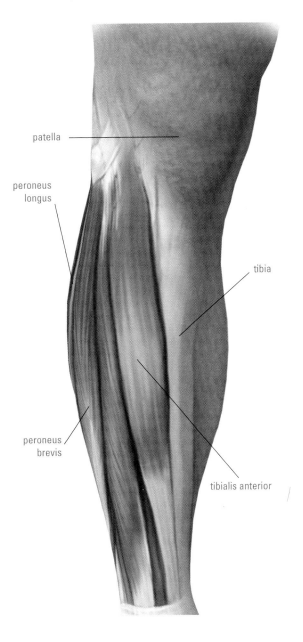

patella

peroneus longus

tibia

peroneus brevis

tibialis anterior

FRONT OF LEGS (CONTINUED)

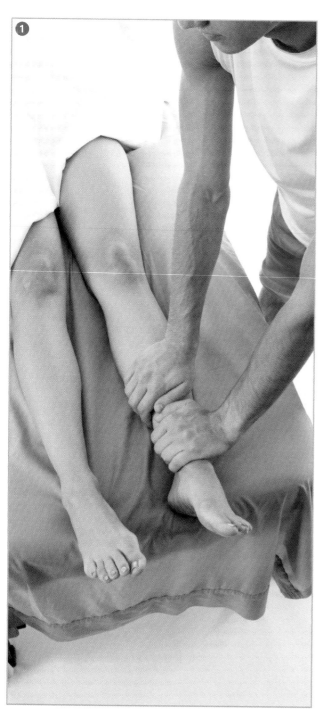

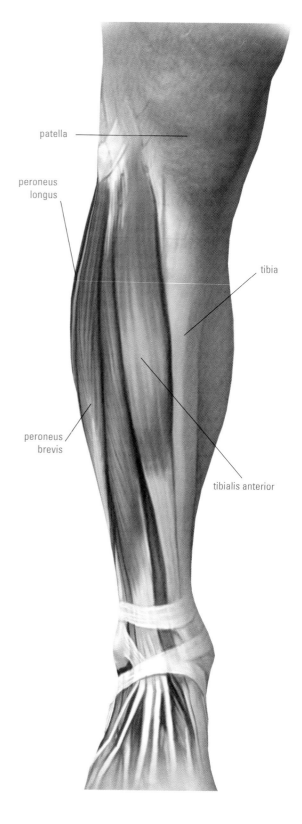

patella

peroneus
longus

tibia

peroneus
brevis

tibialis anterior

①–② Next, rub your subject's leg, back and forth, all the way from the thigh down to the ankles and back up to the thigh.

3 Follow that with compression along the entire leg. Place both hands on your subject's leg and press gently.

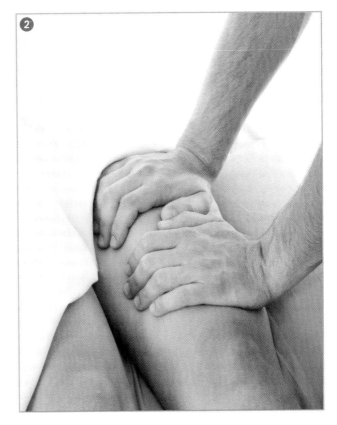

CAUTION

The knee is the largest and most complicated joint in your body. It's also the most fragile, so it's very important that you avoid placing direct pressure on top of the kneecap. Instead, work the sides of the knee.

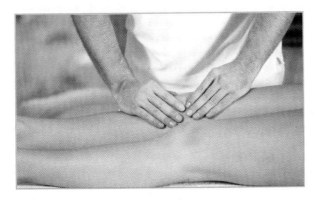

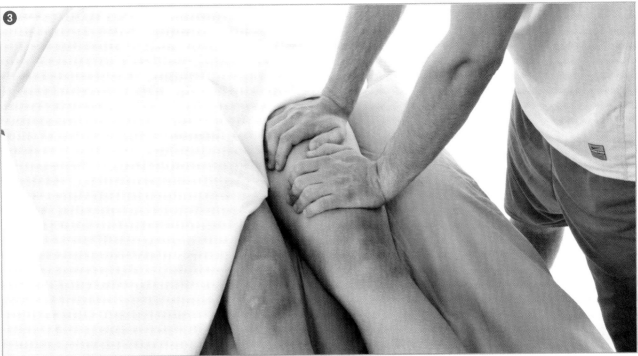

FRONT OF LEGS (CONTINUED)

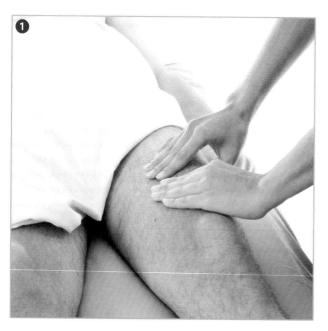

①–② Next, squeeze along the rectus femoris—the muscle on the top of the thigh that runs from the hip to the knee. Its job is to flex the knee and the hip; every time you walk, that muscle works, and so it's worth paying it some extra attention.

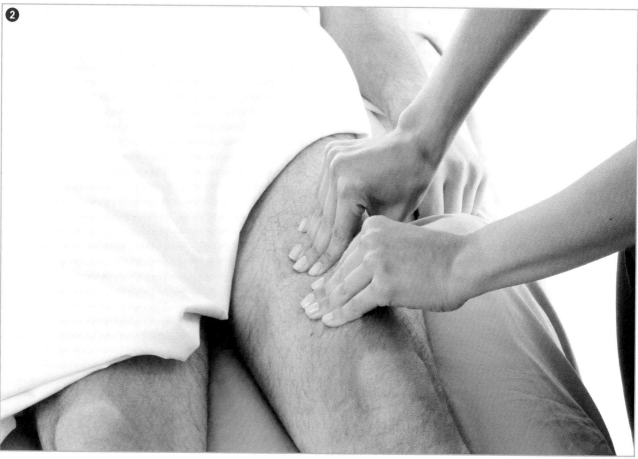

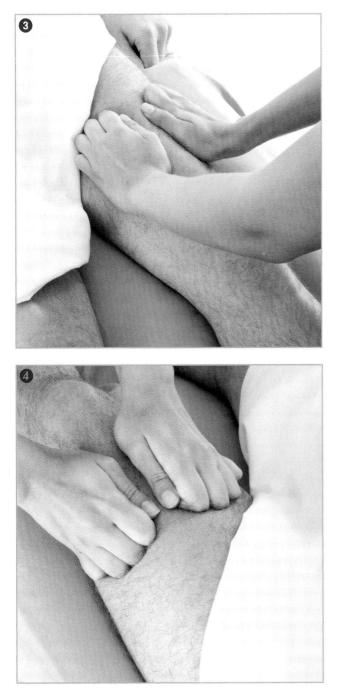

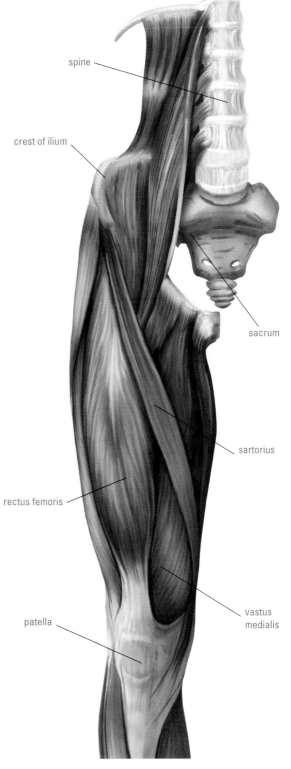

spine

crest of ilium

sacrum

sartorius

rectus femoris

vastus medialis

patella

3–**4** Now, make soft open fists with both your hands and run your knuckles along the rectus femoris. Start at the knee and continue up your subject's leg to his hip.

FRONT OF LEGS (CONTINUED)

1 Make a soft closed fist with one hand and support that hand at the wrist with your other hand. Gently press your fist directly into the rectus femoris, from the knee to the hip.

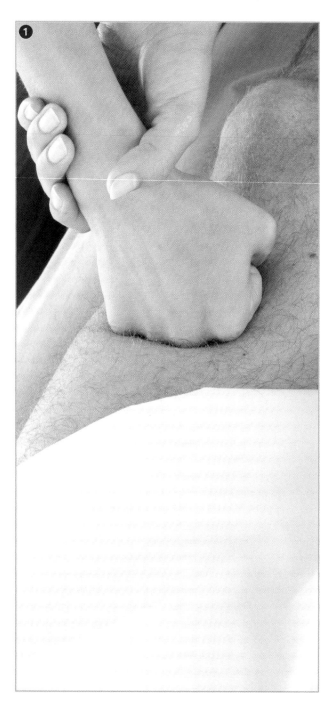

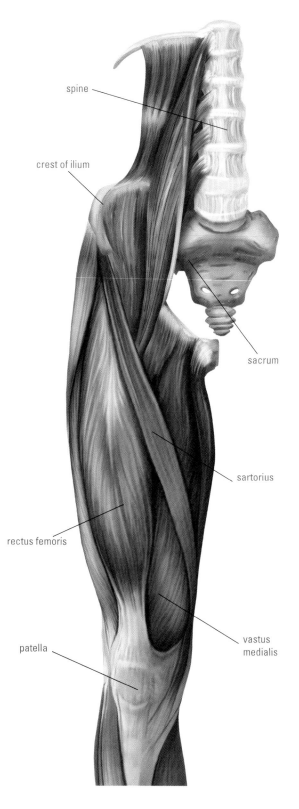

spine

crest of ilium

sacrum

sartorius

rectus femoris

vastus medialis

patella

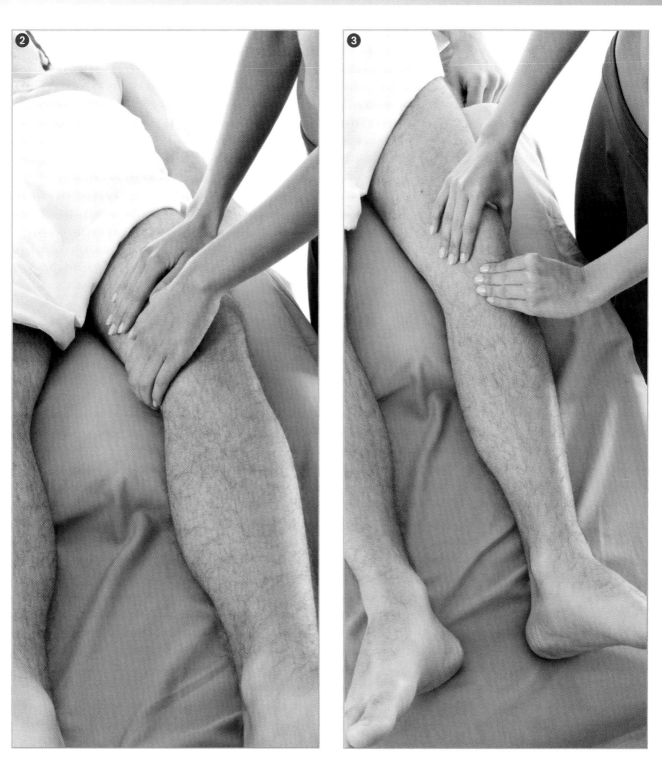

2–**3** Now gently work around the knee, grabbing and squeezing the fleshy part of the leg near the vastus medialis.

FRONT OF LEGS (CONTINUED)

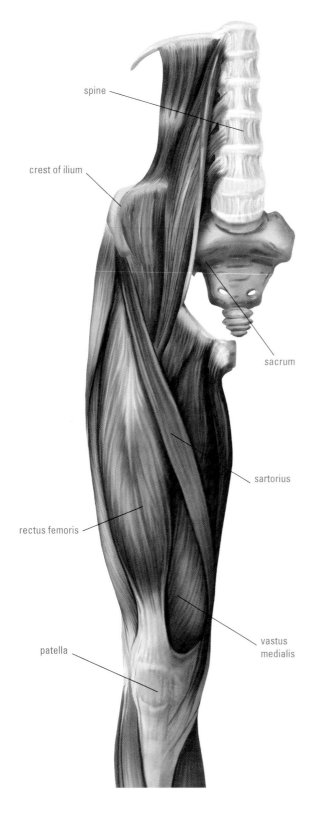

spine

crest of ilium

sacrum

sartorius

rectus femoris

vastus medialis

patella

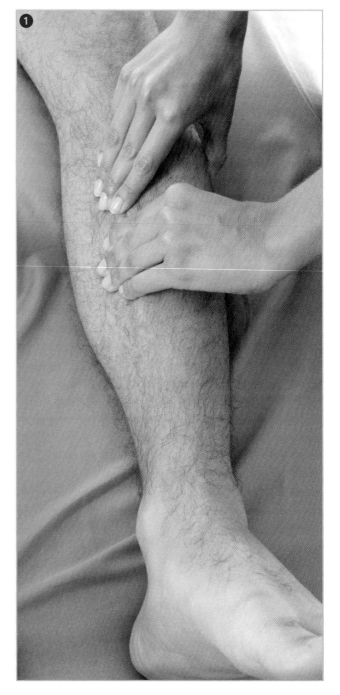

1 Now that the entire leg is well warmed up, grasp the leg with both hands and rub your fingers in small circles. Start at the ankle and work your way up to the upper thigh.

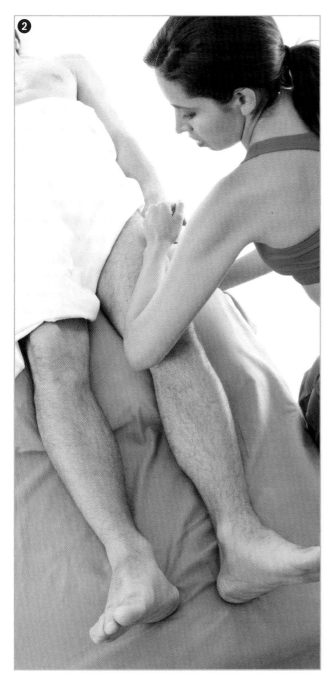

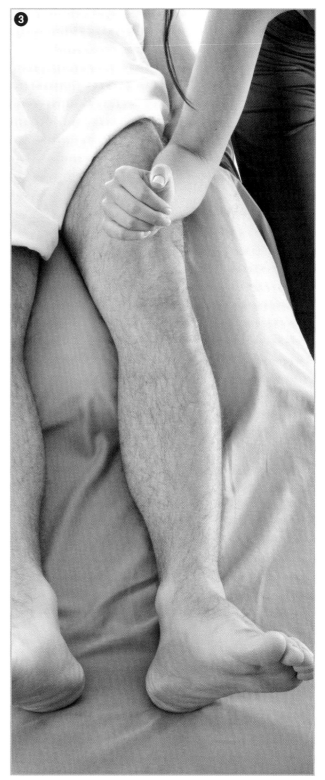

②–③ Finally, use the meaty part of your forearm to press the inside of your subject's thigh, from the knee up as far as is comfortable. Be careful not to bump the knee or put too much pressure on it.

④ UPPER BODY: FRONT

Once you've massaged the lower legs, you'll be moving on to the upper body—first to the abs and then the chest.

Take special care when massaging the abdominal area. It's a very vulnerable spot and one that most people haven't had massaged. Remember, work slowly and gently, and if it turns out to be uncomfortable, you can always skip it and move to the chest or neck and face.

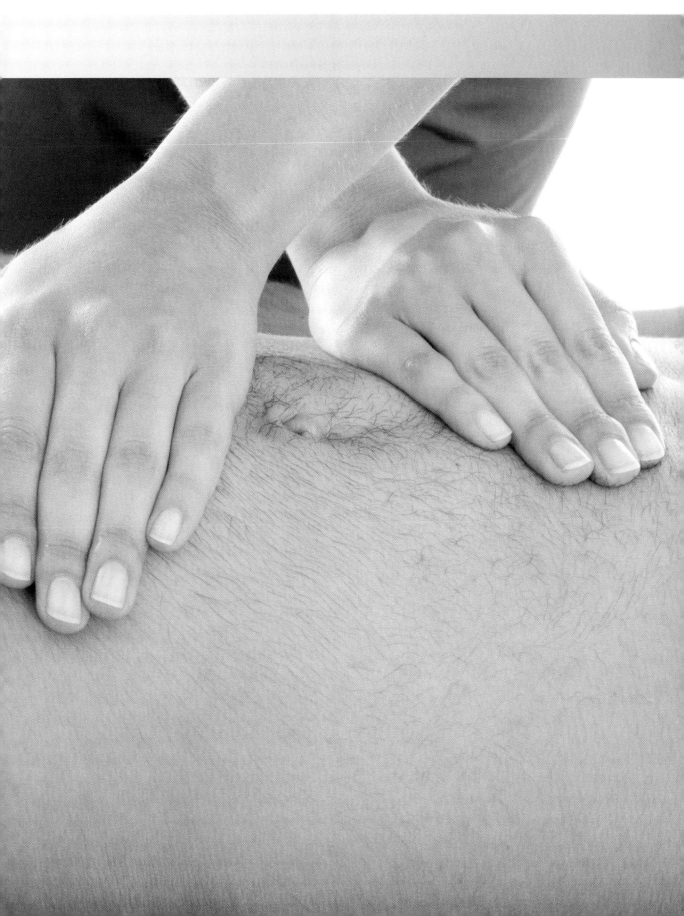

ABS & CHEST

The abdominal muscles (or "abs") are actually made up of four separate muscles: the internal and external obliques, the rectus abdominis, and the transversus abdominis. Together, these muscles help us stand upright, twist, turn, and bend.

Many professional massage therapists don't include ab massage in a full-body massage because it's a soft, vulnerable part of the body, and for some people, having that area worked can bring up feelings and emotions. Always use light, gentle pressure when massaging the abs.

The chest is comprised of two muscles, the pectoralis major and the pectoralis minor. Those muscles allow us to make hugging and pushing motions.

CAUTION

Do not massage someone who is pregnant or who has high blood pressure or gastrointestinal (GI) issues. An ab massage will probably be uncomfortable for someone who has recently had a heavy meal.

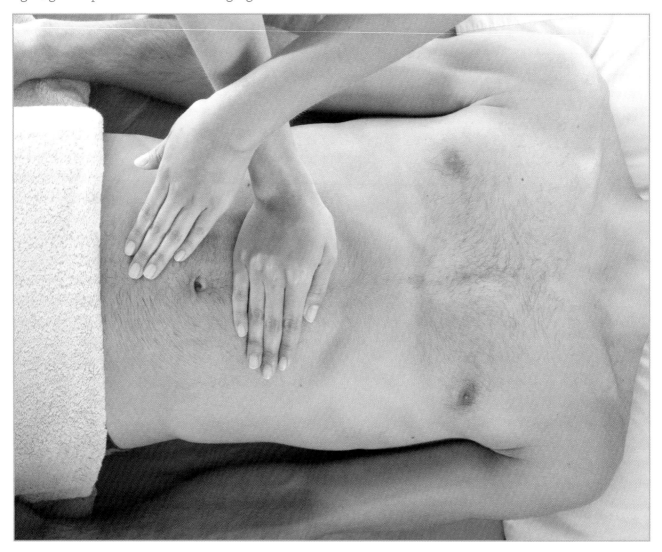

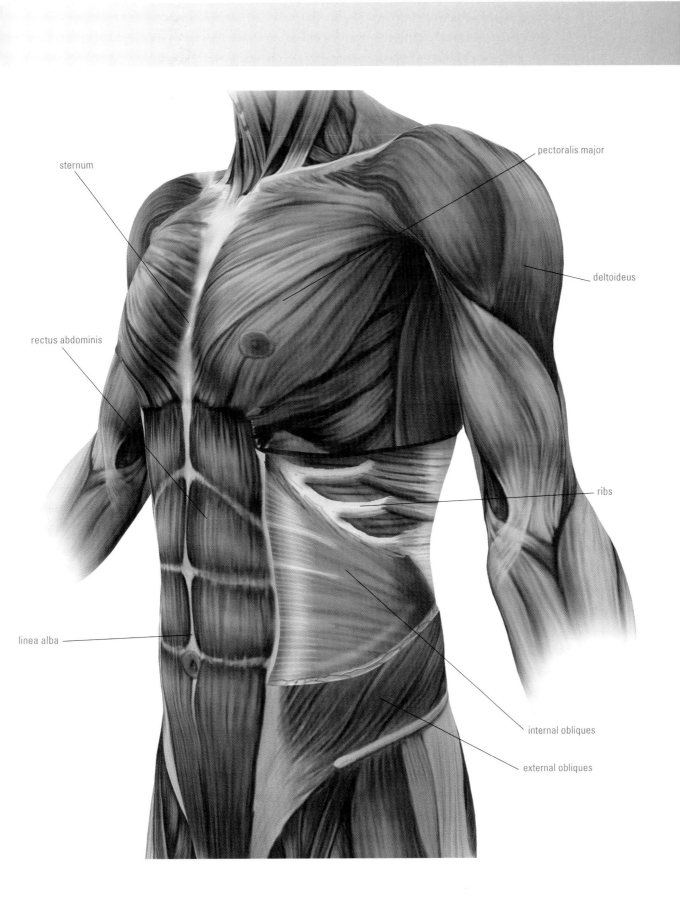

sternum

pectoralis major

deltoideus

rectus abdominis

ribs

linea alba

internal obliques

external obliques

ABS & CHEST (CONTINUED)

1 Begin with the standard effleurage warm-up, but this time use an even gentler touch. Warm the oil in your hands and then ask the person you're massaging to inhale and then exhale. Place your hands on the abdomen on the exhale.

2–3 Place your hands on the abdomen at the nine o'clock and three o'clock positions, with your hands crossed as shown. Next, move your hands in a clockwise direction—the same direction in which digestion takes place. At some point, you'll need to cross your hands again. As you do, make sure to keep at least one hand in contact with the abdomen.

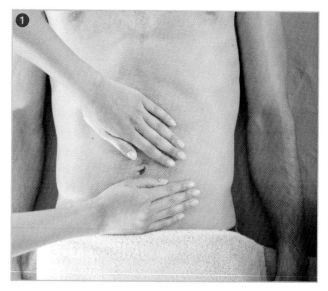

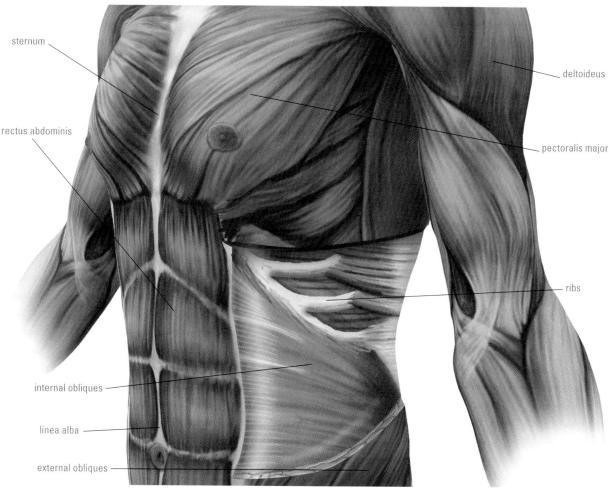

sternum

deltoideus

rectus abdominis

pectoralis major

ribs

internal obliques

linea alba

external obliques

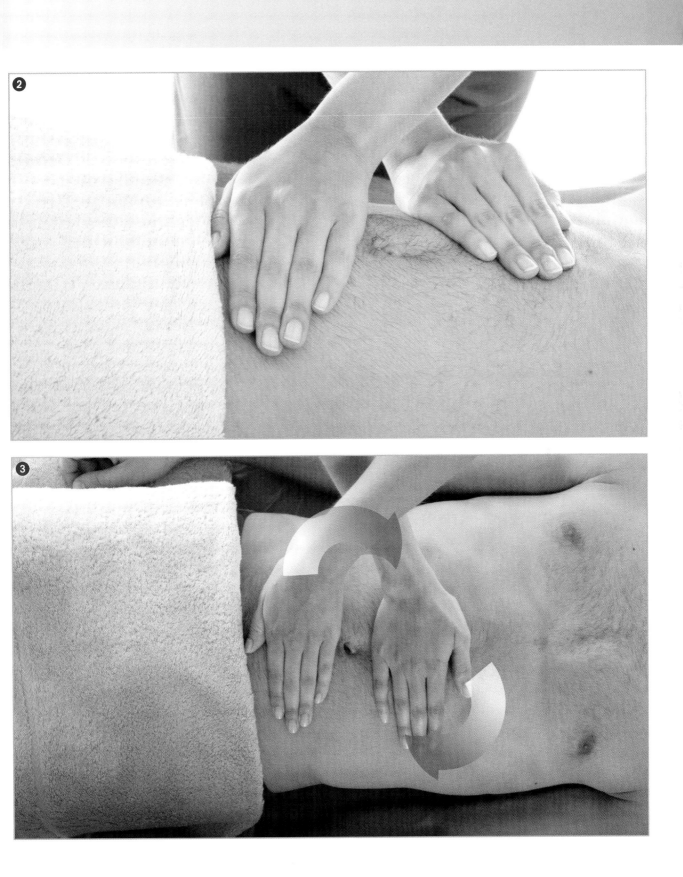

ABS & CHEST (CONTINUED)

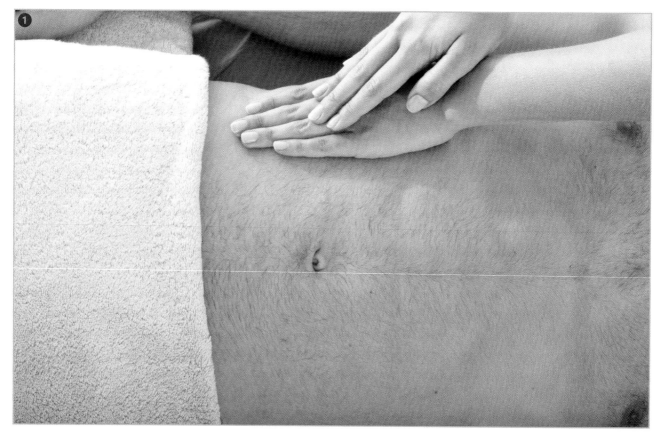

❶ Next, place one hand atop the other and apply gentle pressure around the area between the bottom of the rib cage and the top of the pelvic bone.

❷ Keeping your hands in the same posture, apply gentle pressure along each side of the linea alba—the vertical line that separates the left and right rectus abdominis muscles.

❸–❹ Now, rake the ribs as you did in the face-down position—make a "claw" shape with your hands and place your fingertips between the ribs. Gently pull your hands upward, toward the linea alba. Repeat several times on each side of the body.

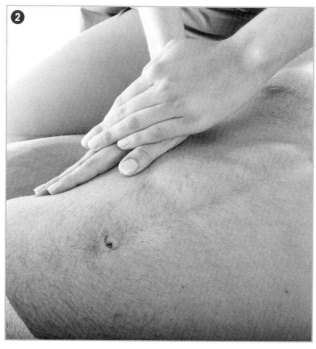

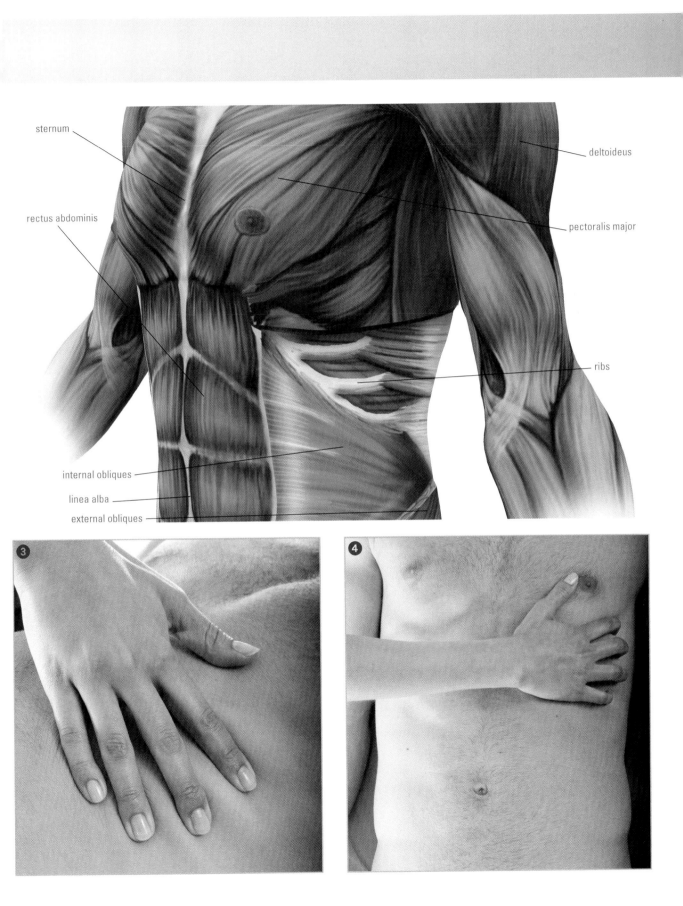

sternum

deltoideus

rectus abdominis

pectoralis major

ribs

internal obliques

linea alba

external obliques

ABS & CHEST (CONTINUED)

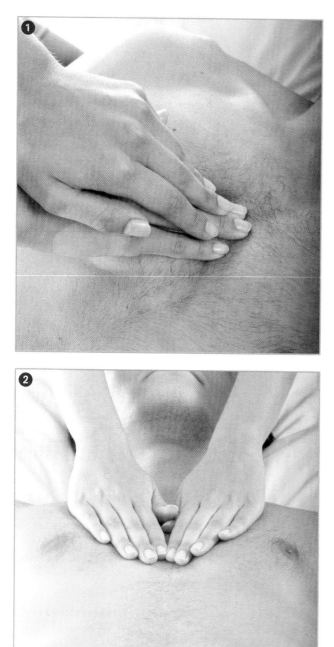

3–4 Now place one hand on each clavicle and, starting at the sternum, massage in a circle around the pectorals, from the inside to the outside. Keep both hands flat at all times.

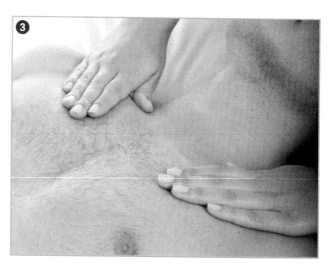

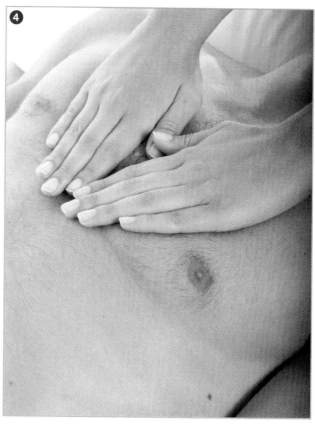

1–2 Next, place one hand atop the other so that the bottom hand's fingers are supported by the top hand's, and gently massage the sternum. Do not press directly on the xiphoid process— the piece of bone at the tip of the sternum— because it could fracture.

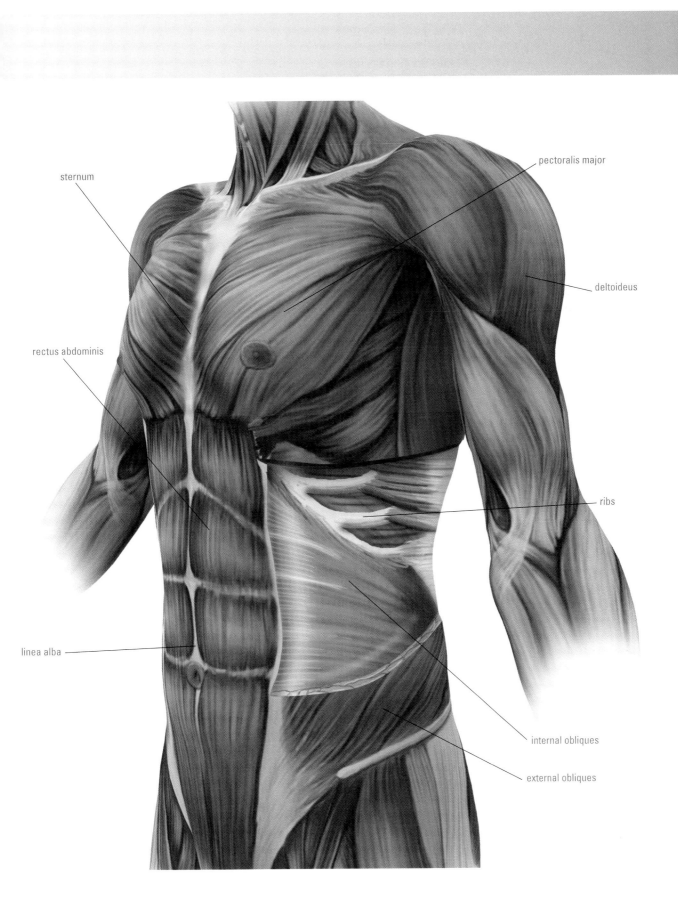

sternum

pectoralis major

deltoideus

rectus abdominis

ribs

linea alba

internal obliques

external obliques

ABS & CHEST (CONTINUED)

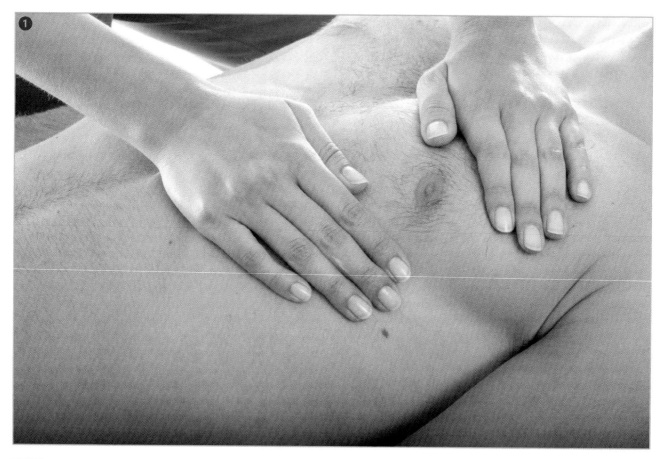

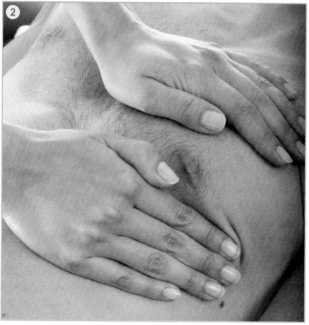

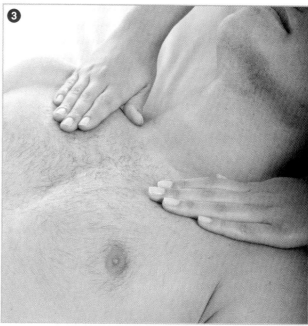

1–**2** Massage around the pecs again, this time starting with your hands as shown. Instead of allowing your hands to glide along the skin, move the skin and massage and squeeze the muscle beneath.

3 Next place one hand on each clavicle (or collarbone) at the shoulder edge so that your thumb is above the bone and the fingers rest below it. Squeezing very slightly, run your fingertips along the clavicle toward the sternum.

CAUTION

When you're massaging around the clavicle, be very gentle and do not press too hard. This is an area with many nerves and blood vessels.

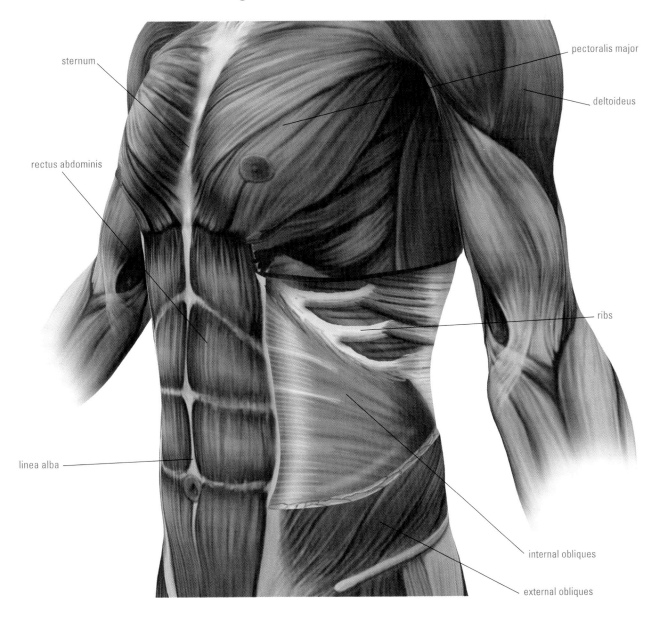

sternum

pectoralis major

deltoideus

rectus abdominis

ribs

linea alba

internal obliques

external obliques

ABS & CHEST (CONTINUED)

Tight pectoral muscles pull the neck forward, so in order to look straight ahead, the upper shoulder and neck muscles have to contract more and work harder to keep the head up, and that causes pain in the upper shoulders and neck. This next stroke will help loosen the pectoral muscles.

Hold the left wrist as shown, making sure that the left arm remains parallel to the body at all times.

❶ Make a soft fist with the left hand and place it under the clavicle, close to the sternum.

❷–**❹** Now slide your fist toward the armpit while at the same time moving the left arm toward the head, keeping it parallel with the body.

Repeat, using the heel of your hand instead of a soft fist.

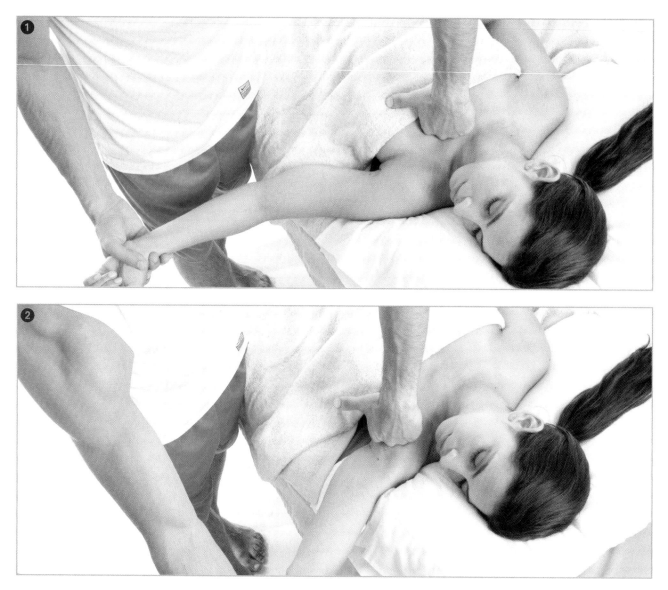

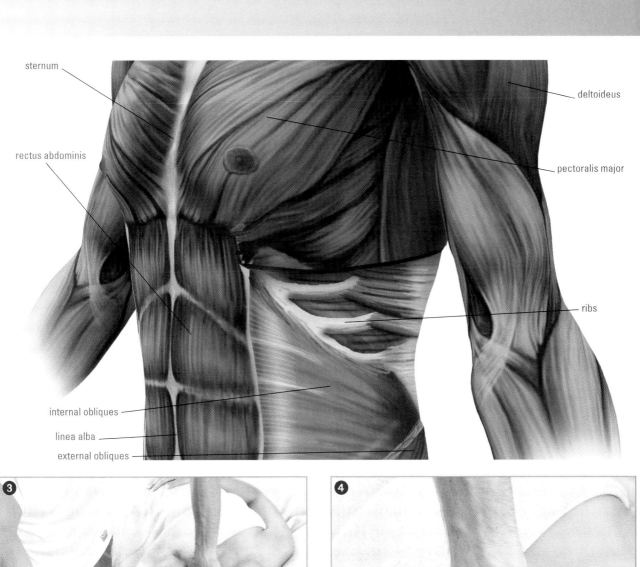

sternum

deltoideus

rectus abdominis

pectoralis major

ribs

internal obliques

linea alba

external obliques

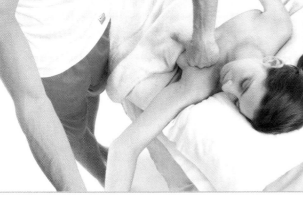

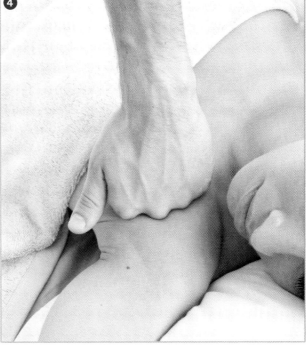

CAUTION

The amount of breast tissue will determine how much pressure you can use. Check in with the person you're massaging.

ARMS & SHOULDERS

We use our arms and shoulders in so many ways each day that most people probably don't give them much thought. Swinging a tennis racket or softball bat, sitting at a desk typing, cleaning around the house, and holding a cell phone against your head are all activities that involve your arms and shoulders. And because we do use them so frequently, arms and shoulders almost always benefit from massage.

CAUTION

- There are three primary nerves in the arm. One of them, the ulnar nerve, runs from the clavicle (collarbone) to the little finger. The ulnar nerve is almost completely unprotected where it runs over the elbow, and that's why hitting your "funny bone" is so painful. What you're actually hitting is that nerve. That's just one reason to be careful when massaging around the elbow and shoulder joints.

- A second reason is that care needs to be taken around joints in general. It can be easy to force a joint beyond its range of motion, so always move the limbs gently and slowly.

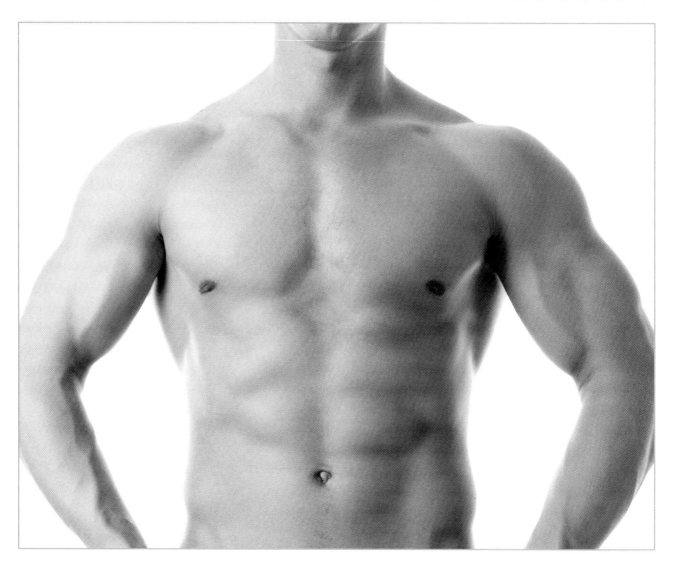

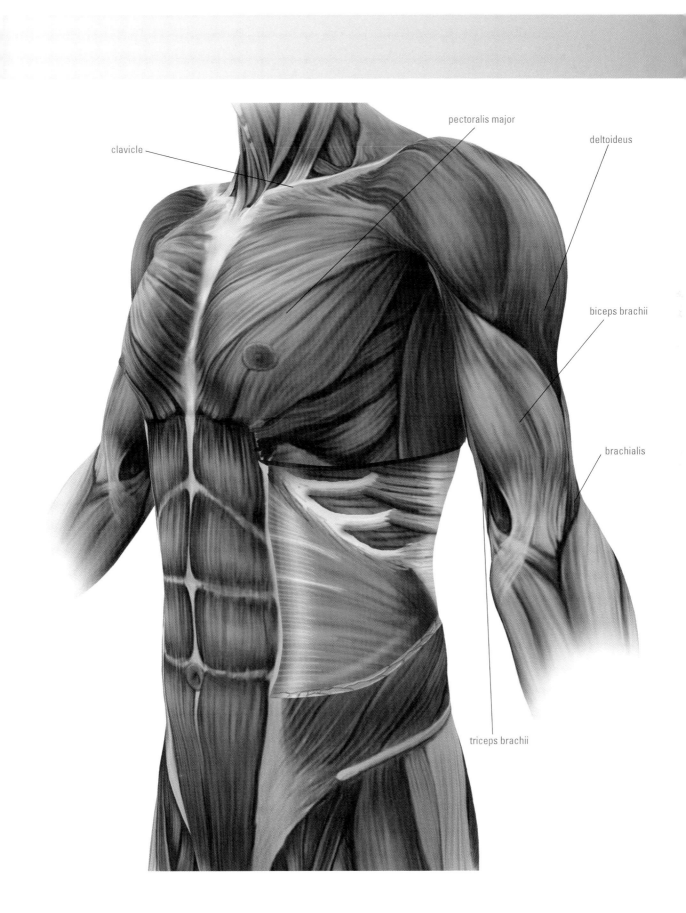

clavicle

pectoralis major

deltoideus

biceps brachii

brachialis

triceps brachii

ARMS & SHOULDERS

①–③ Begin by warming the oil in your hands and then applying gentle strokes (effleurage) from the wrist to the shoulder to warm up the arm and get the blood flowing.

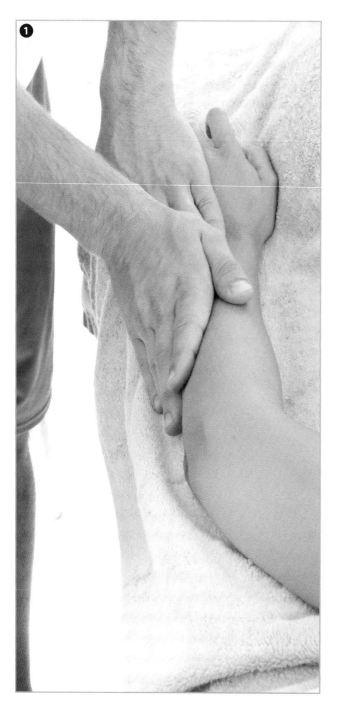

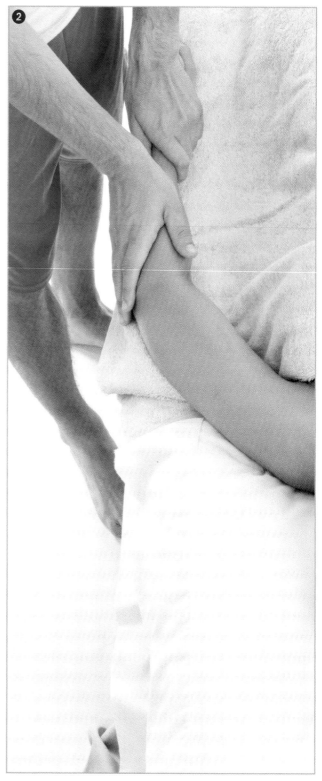

(CONTINUED)

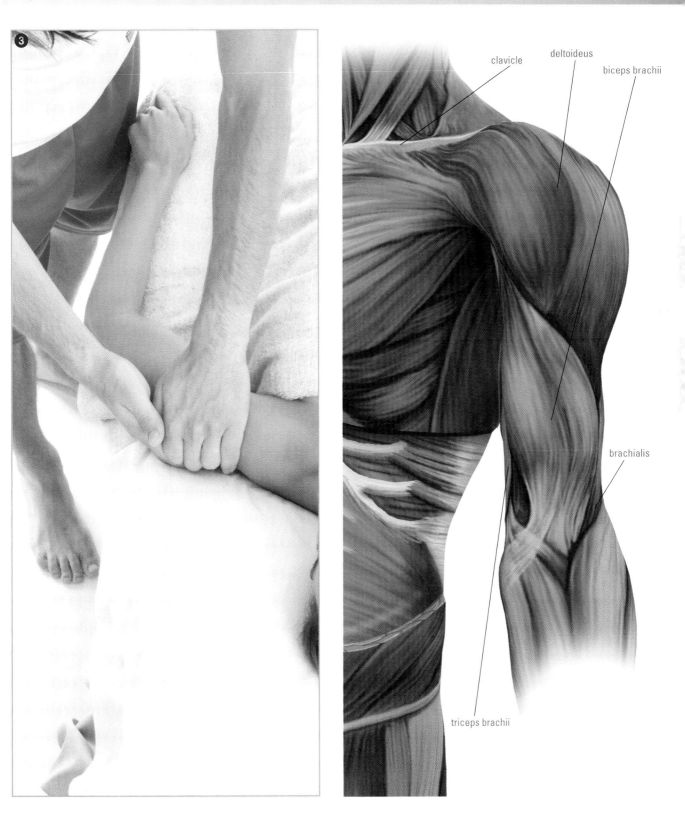

ARMS & SHOULDERS

①–③ Next, place your fingertips on the clavicle. Applying gentle pressure, slide your fingers from the collarbone outward to the armpit. This feels very nice and also moves lymph toward the lymph nodes.

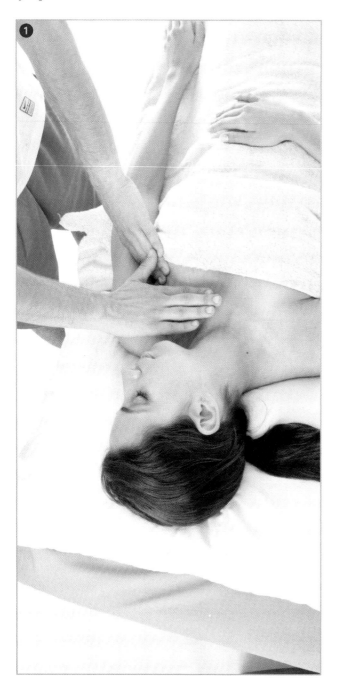

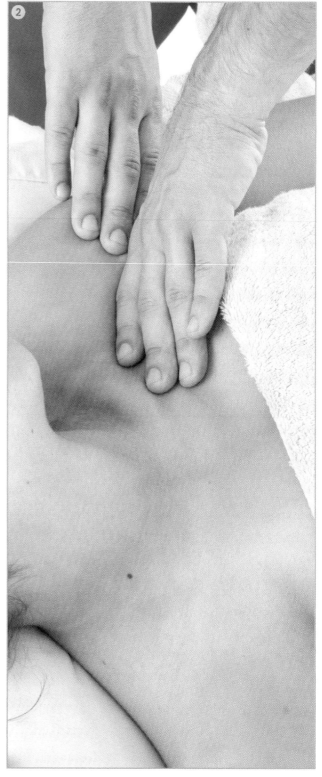

(CONTINUED)

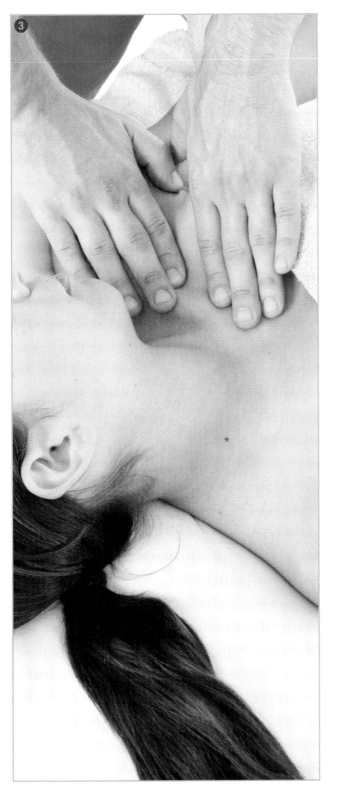

MASSAGE TIPS

Lymph is a clear fluid that circulates through the body collecting foreign microbes such as those that cause and result from infections. Increasing lymph flow helps clear those toxins from the body. In addition, massage has been found to improve the range of motion of joints, relax muscles, and trigger the release of endorphins—the body's "feel-good" chemicals.

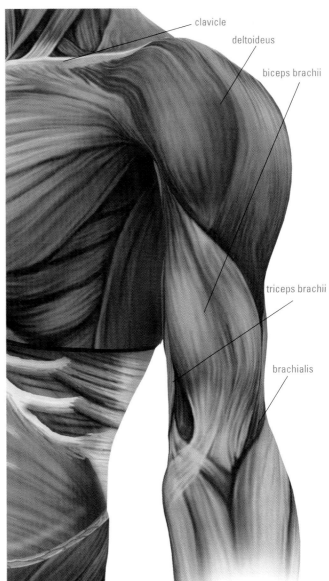

clavicle

deltoideus

biceps brachii

triceps brachii

brachialis

ARMS & SHOULDERS

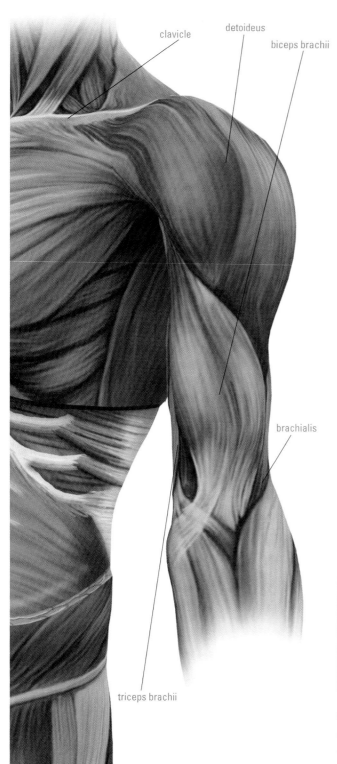

clavicle

detoideus

biceps brachii

brachialis

triceps brachii

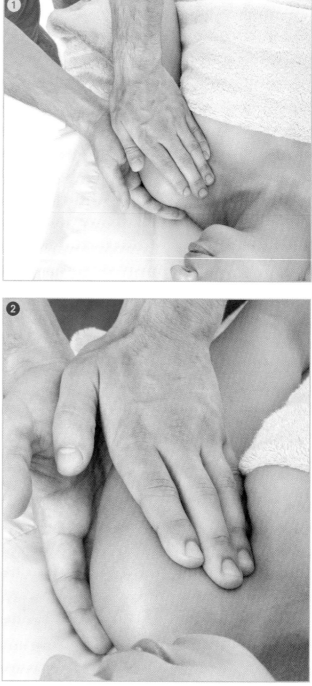

1–**2** Place your hands around the shoulder (this is called "cupping" the shoulder) and rub the skin back and forth.

(CONTINUED)

3–**5** Now, grasp the biceps as shown and squeeze with alternating hands along the muscle from the shoulder to the wrist. Take care not to squeeze the elbow joint.

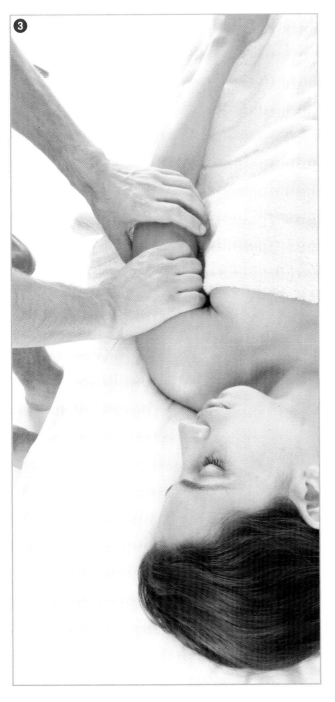

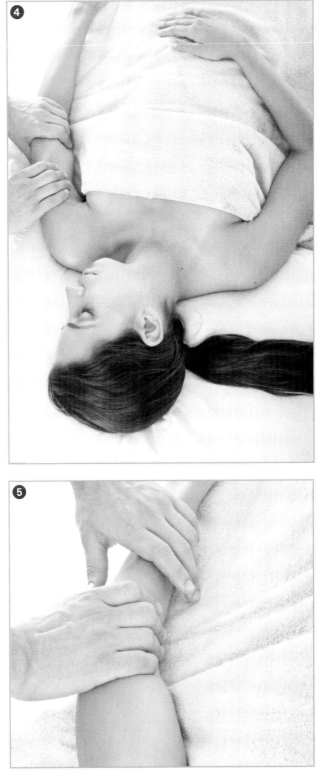

ARMS & SHOULDERS

①–③ Gently hold the left hand with your right hand as shown—hold the hand rather than the wrist. Place your left hand on the left triceps. While gently rotating the arm toward you, rub the triceps muscle away from you.

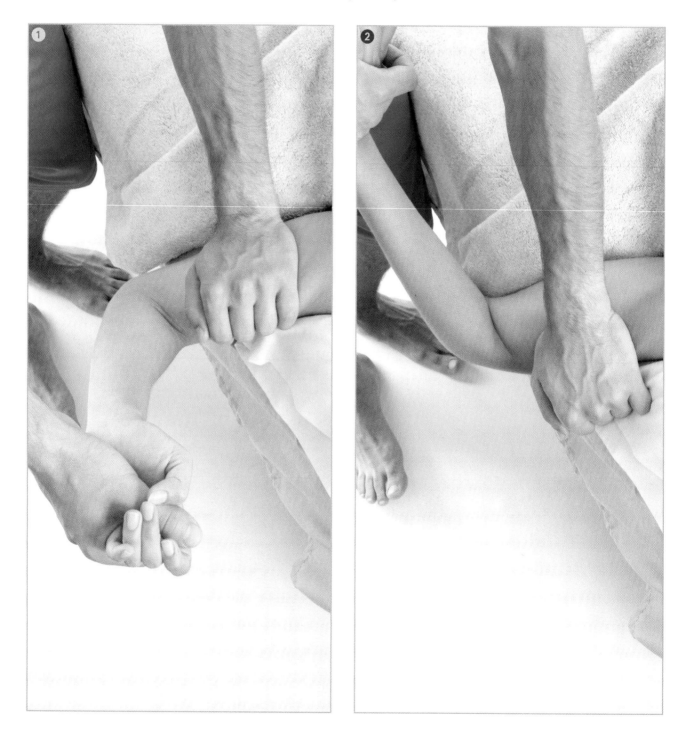

(CONTINUED)

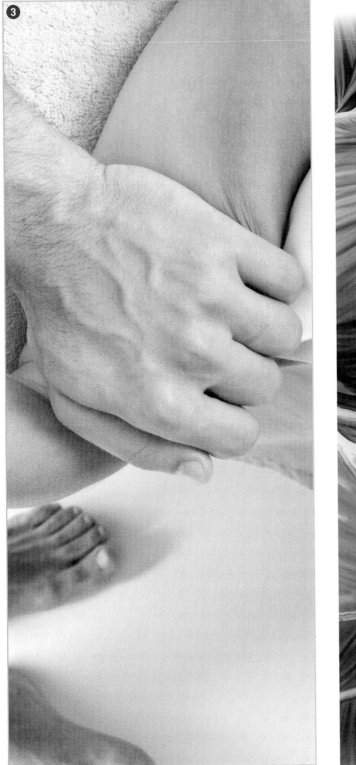

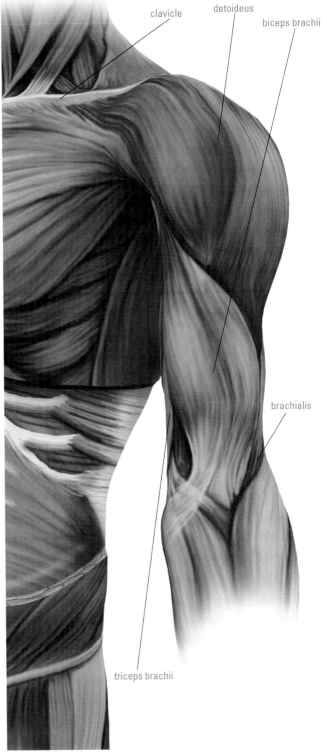

clavicle

detoideus

biceps brachii

brachialis

triceps brachii

ARMS & SHOULDERS

1–**3** Next, you will strip the sides of the bra-chioradialis, the largest muscle of the forearm. Place your hand on the brachioradialis as shown, as if you were going to "pinch" it, and then slide your hand toward the elbow, applying gentle pressure.

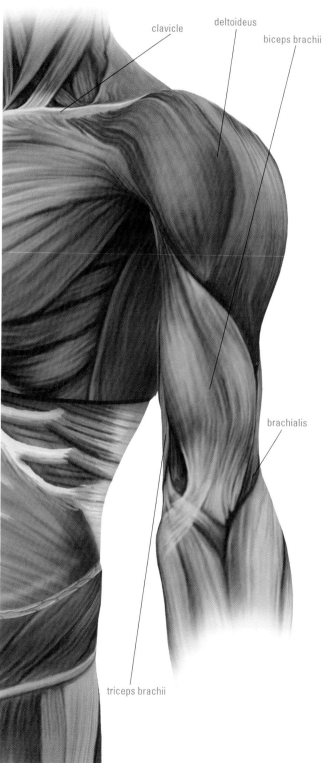

clavicle

deltoideus

biceps brachii

brachialis

triceps brachii

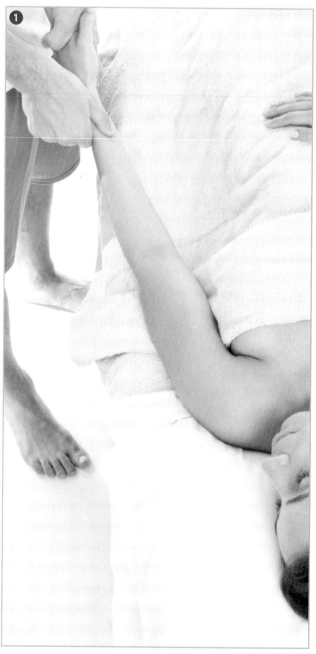

(CONTINUED)

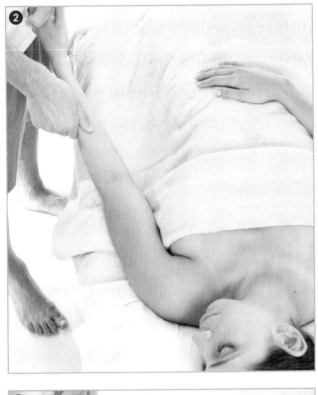

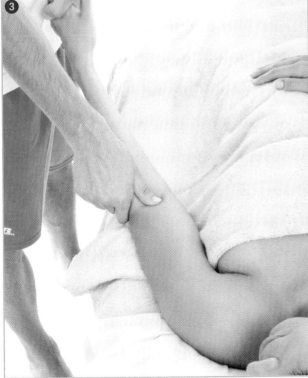

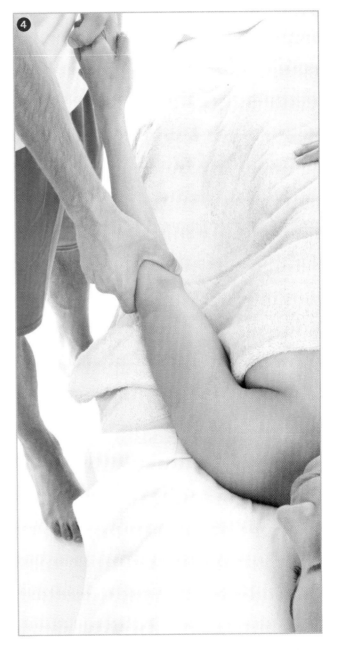

4 Repeat the motion, this time using the web of skin between the thumb and index finger to strip the muscle.

Once you have completed the shoulder and arm massage on one side, repeat with the opposite arm and shoulder.

HANDS

Among the most intricate and complicated parts of the body, our hands make us unique in the animal kingdom. Our fully opposable thumbs allow us to hold and use tools and other items. And because our hands—along with their twenty-seven bones and twenty-five muscles—are almost always active, it's not surprising that a hand massage feels so good.

CAUTION

Take care massaging the hand when a person has arthritis. Be gentle and ask for feedback.

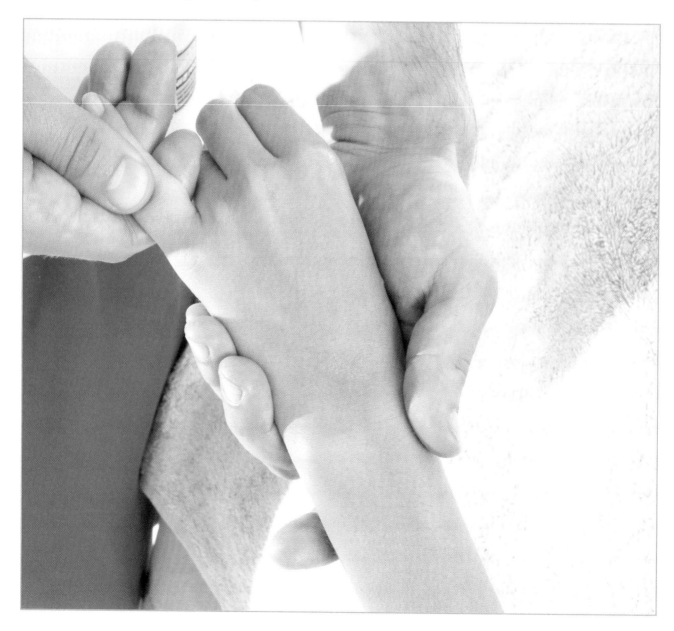

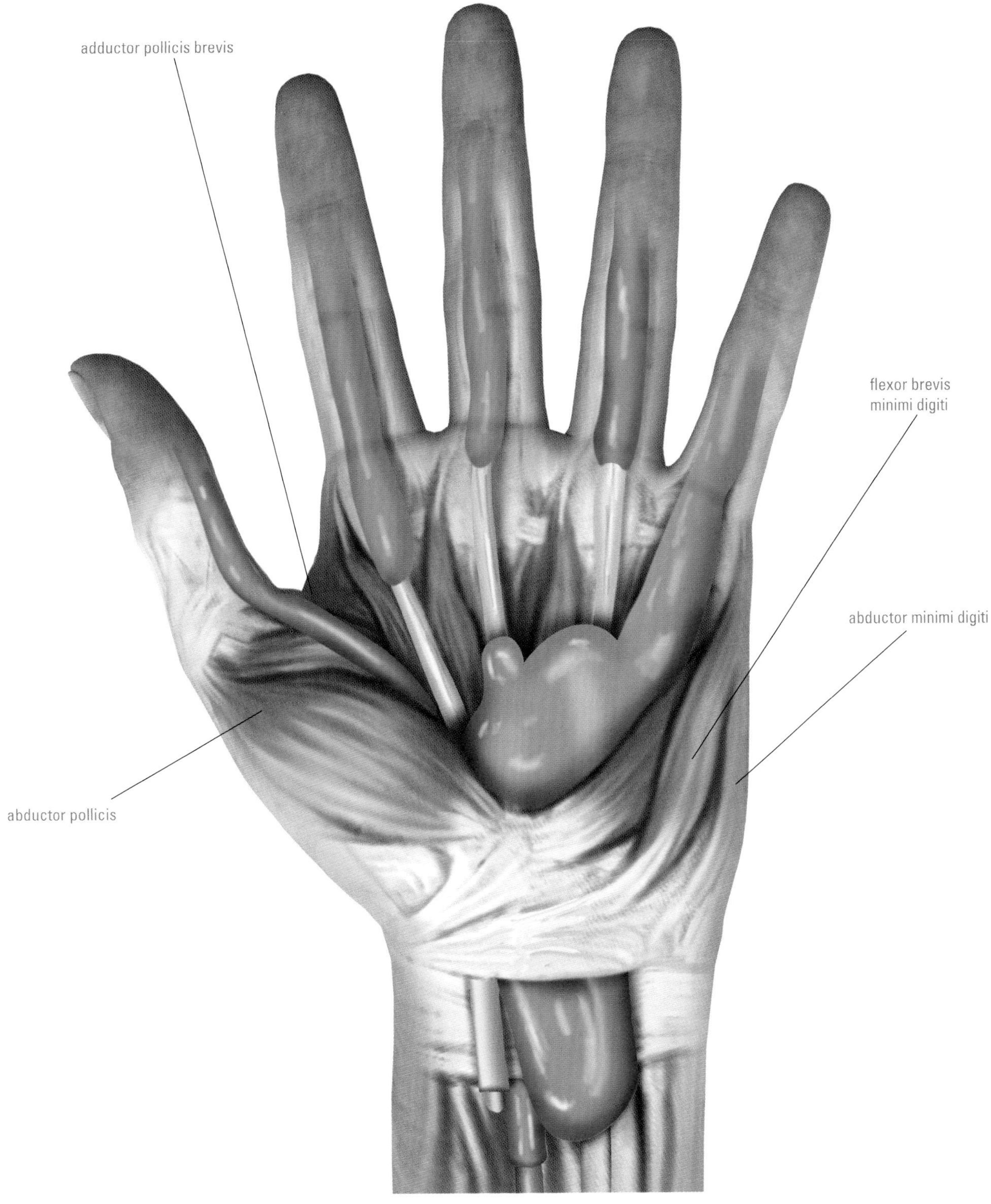

adductor pollicis brevis

flexor brevis
minimi digiti

abductor minimi digiti

abductor pollicis

HANDS (CONTINUED)

1–**2** Start by holding and supporting the hand as shown. With your thumbs, gently work the area where the arm and wrist meet, between the carpals and the radius and ulna.

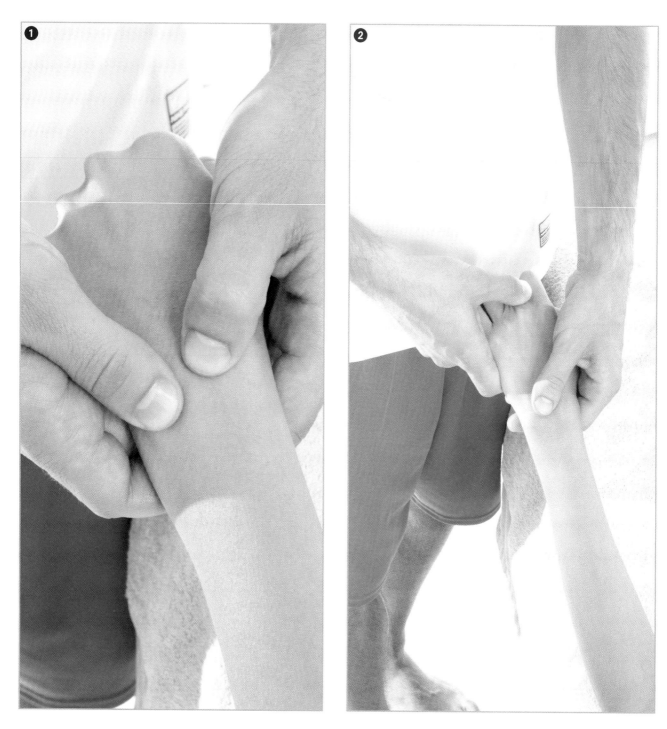

adductor pollicis brevis

flexor brevis
minimi digiti

abductor minimi digiti

abductor pollicis

HANDS (CONTINUED)

1–**3** Next, hold one of the hands as shown, with one of your thumbs on the base of your subject's thumb and your other thumb at the base of your subject's little finger. Keep your subject's thumb and little finger between the first two fingers of each of your hands. Massage the palm of the hand with your thumbs, running them from the heel of the hand to the base of the fingers and then in circles.

4 Now, turn over the hand and massage each finger, squeezing along its length.

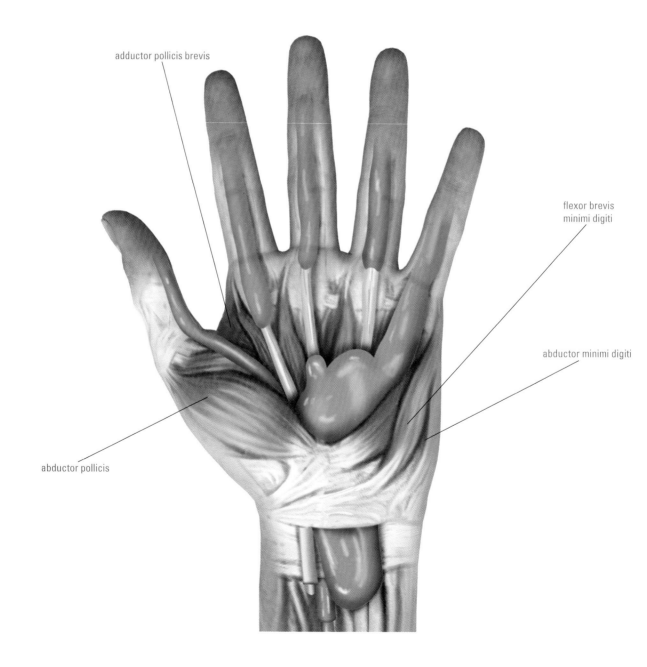

adductor pollicis brevis

flexor brevis minimi digiti

abductor minimi digiti

abductor pollicis

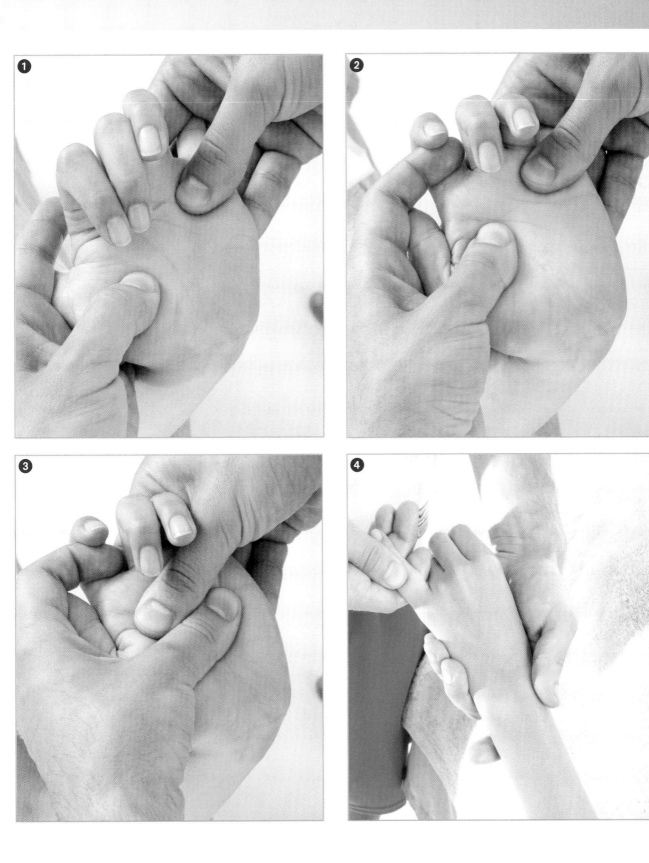

HANDS (CONTINUED)

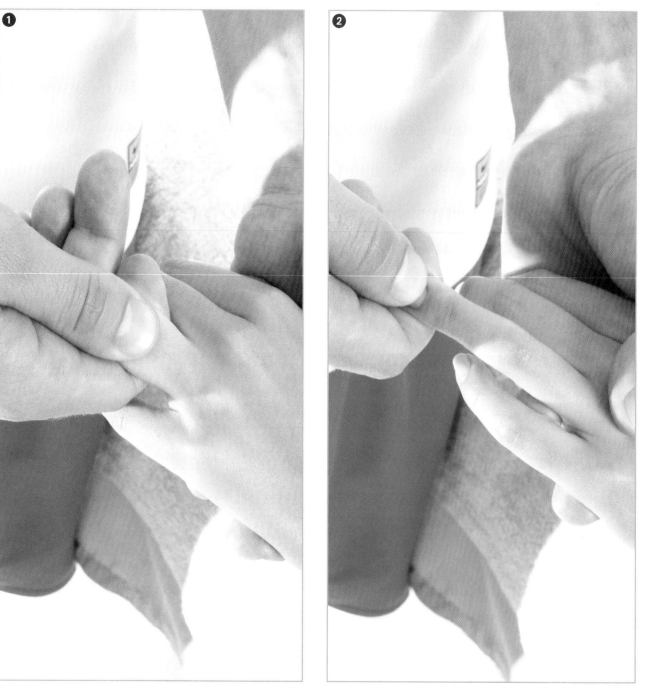

❶ Repeat the finger massage, this time also very gently twisting each finger after you've squeezed each along its length. Be sure to support the hand above and below the wrist joint.

❷ Finally, very gently squeeze each finger at the base of the fingernail.

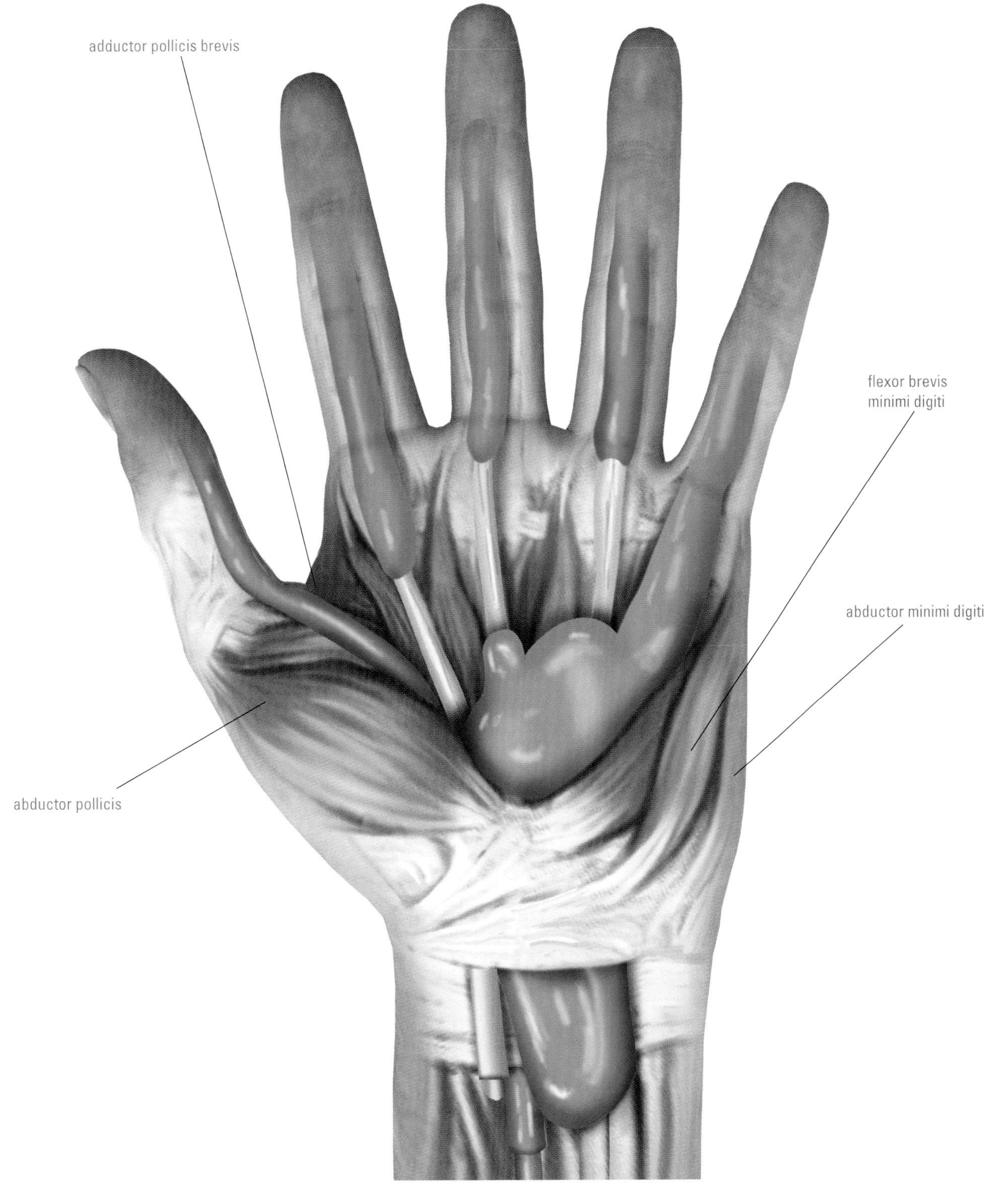

adductor pollicis brevis

flexor brevis minimi digiti

abductor minimi digiti

abductor pollicis

⑤ THE HEAD

The last stop on the full-body massage is the head. In this section, you'll begin by working the neck—an area in which most people carry at least some muscle tension. From there, you'll move on to the face and then the top of the head. Finally, the section ends with some advice about how to proceed after the massage is finished.

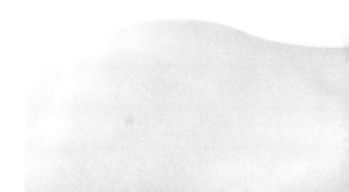

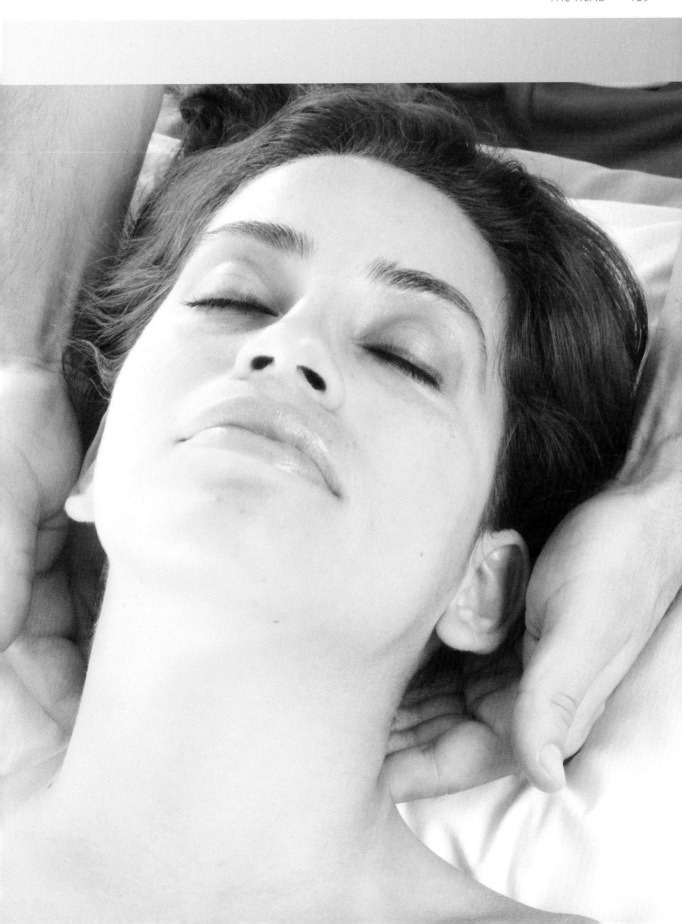

NECK

Most of us carry some tension in our necks. When the muscles of the neck are tight, the result can be a tension headache. Tension in the neck can be caused by stress, poor posture while sitting at a computer, even sleeping in awkward positions. Regular massage of the area will go a long way toward eliminating the problem.

CAUTION

The neck is an area rich in nerves and blood vessels, and so great care must be taken when massaging there.

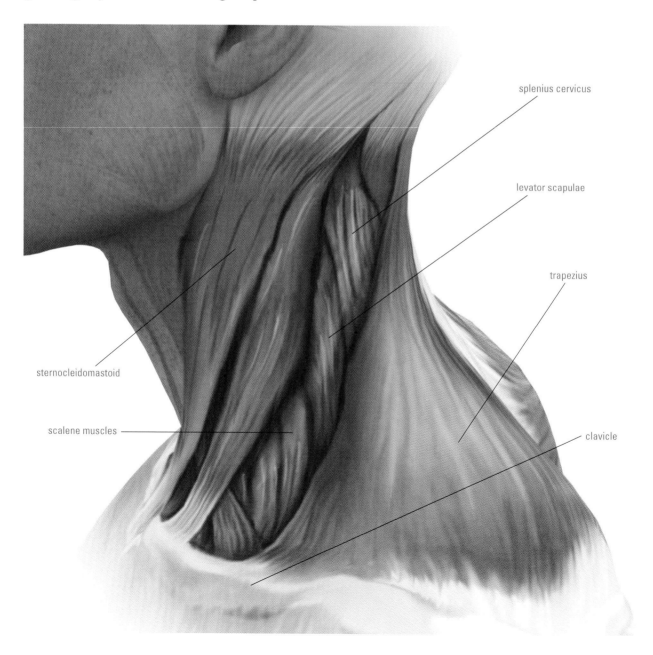

splenius cervicus

levator scapulae

trapezius

sternocleidomastoid

scalene muscles

clavicle

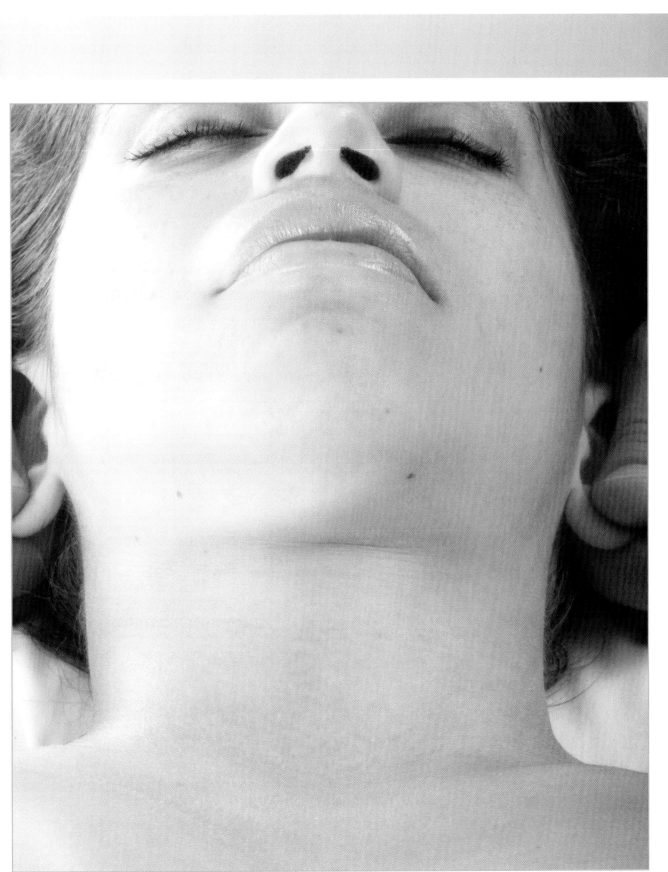

NECK (CONTINUED)

1–**2** To begin the neck massage, make a soft fist and place it behind the sternocleidomastoid (also known as the SCM). Pressing very gently, run your fist from just below the ear to the upper shoulder.

CAUTION

The person you're massaging may ask you to press hard when you do this stroke, but don't—especially if the person is over fifty-five years of age, because you can loosen plaque in the artery that runs to the brain.

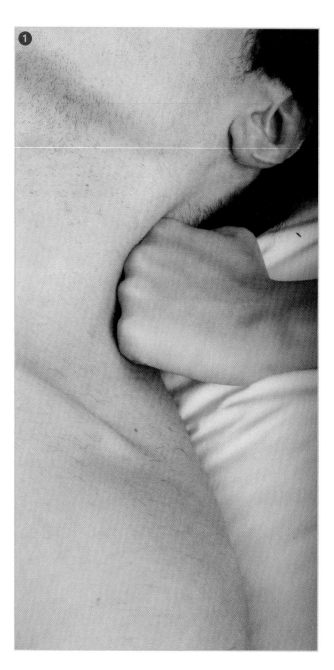

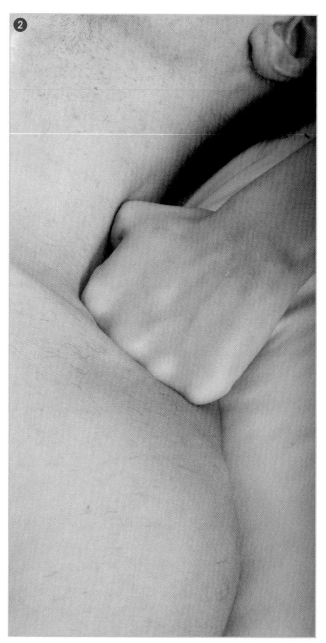

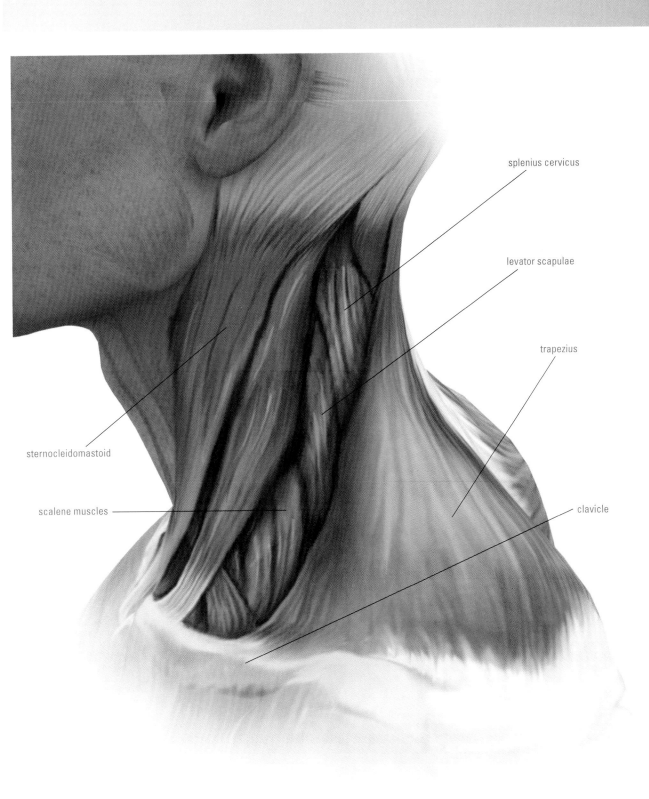

splenius cervicus

levator scapulae

trapezius

sternocleidomastoid

scalene muscles

clavicle

NECK (CONTINUED)

①–② Now repeat the same motion, but rather than using your fist to massage the area, open your hand a bit and run your first set of knuckles down the side of the neck. Again, press gently, and behind the SCM.

③–⑤ Repeat the motion once again, this time using the web of skin between your thumb and index finger to massage the side of the neck.

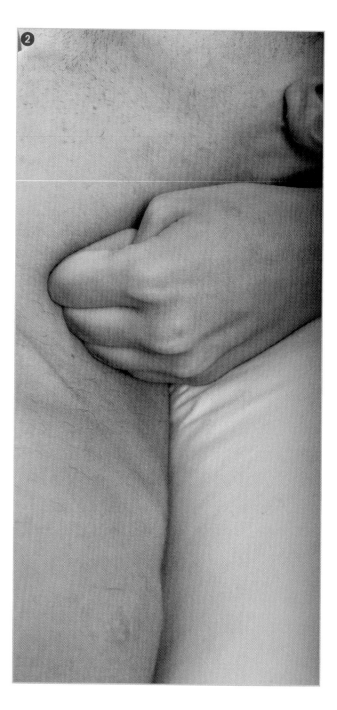

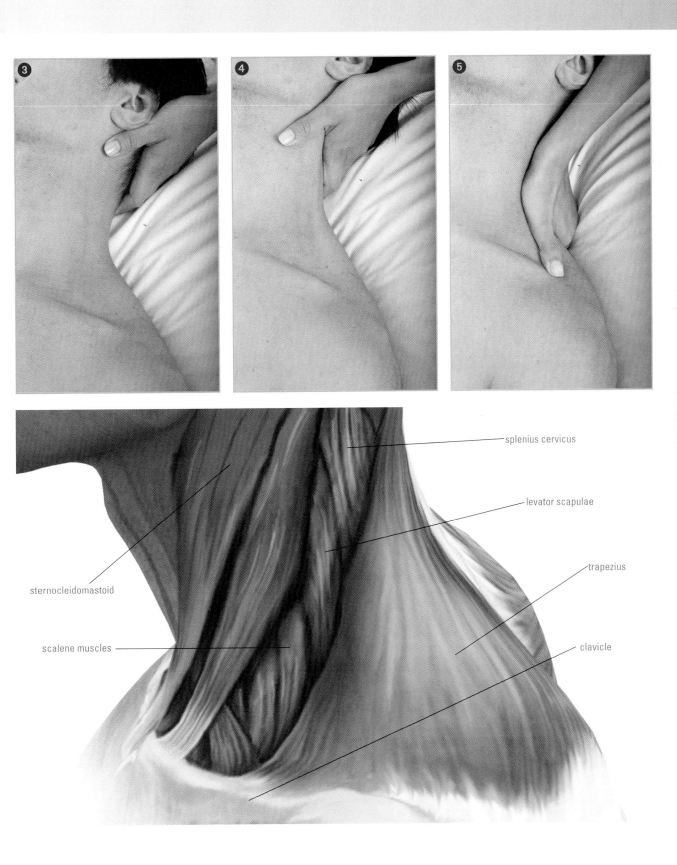

splenius cervicus

levator scapulae

trapezius

sternocleidomastoid

clavicle

scalene muscles

FACE

Most people don't realize how much tension they hold in their facial muscles until they have a massage. There are forty-three muscles in the face; massaging them can reduce tension and increase circulation. Some people believe that regular facial massage reduces wrinkles and makes the skin look younger. Even without those potential benefits, a facial massage is very pleasurable.

Before you massage the face, make sure to use a hand sanitizer or wash your hands—remember, you recently massaged the person's feet.

Some people don't care for massage oil on their face; some have enough natural oil on their skin. So before you warm the oil in your hands, check.

Also keep in mind that while you're massaging the face and head, you'll be resting your hands on your subject's hair, so ask ahead of time if they mind having oil in their hair.

Let your subject know when you're starting, so they won't be surprised when you place your hands on their face.

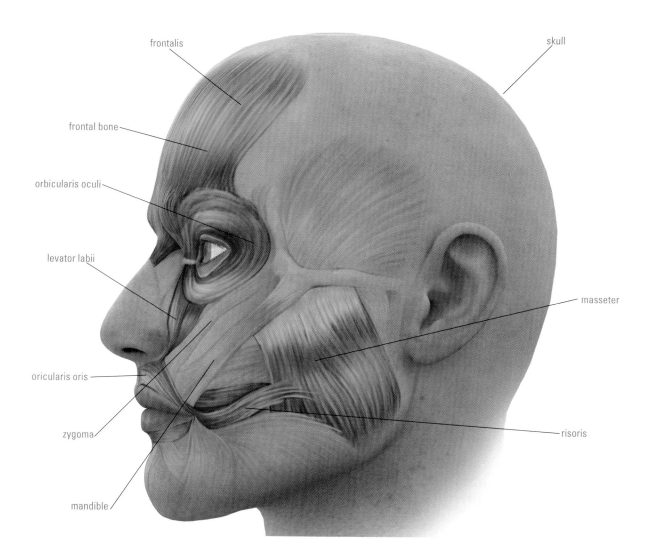

frontalis

skull

frontal bone

orbicularis oculi

levator labii

masseter

oricularis oris

zygoma

risoris

mandible

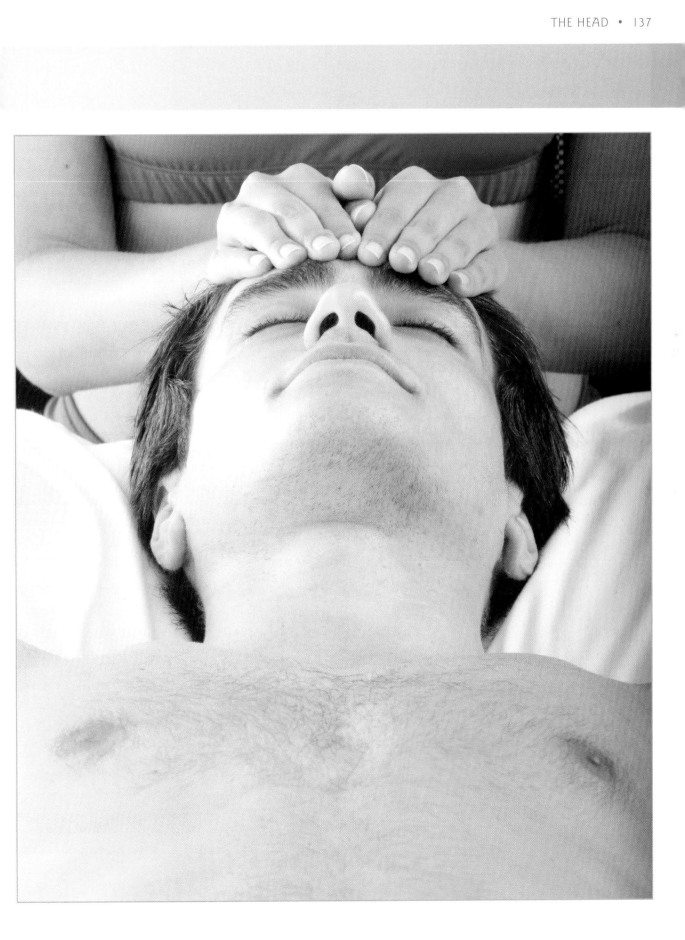

FACE (CONTINUED)

①–② Softly place your fingertips on the fore-head. Gently glide them along the brow to the temple and back again.

③ Continue with that same motion, this time continuing beyond the temples until you're nearly at the ears, then back again.

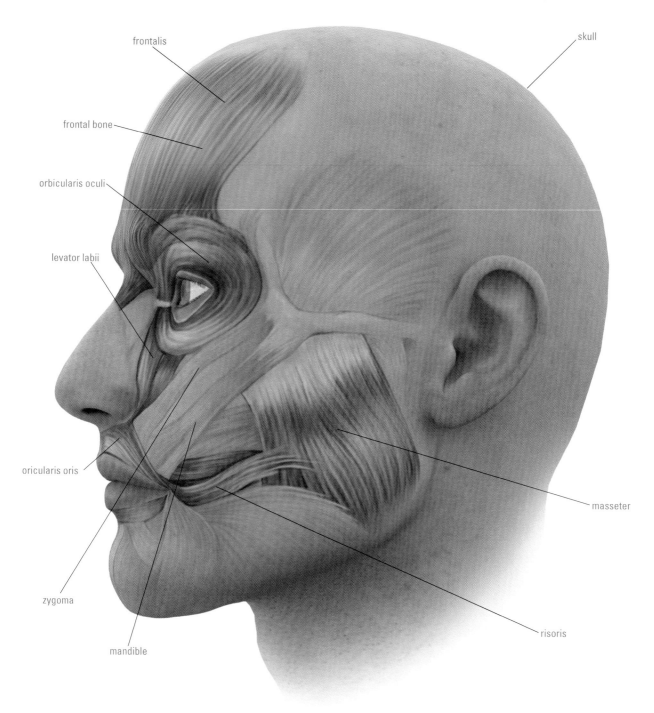

frontalis

skull

frontal bone

orbicularis oculi

levator labii

oricularis oris

masseter

zygoma

risoris

mandible

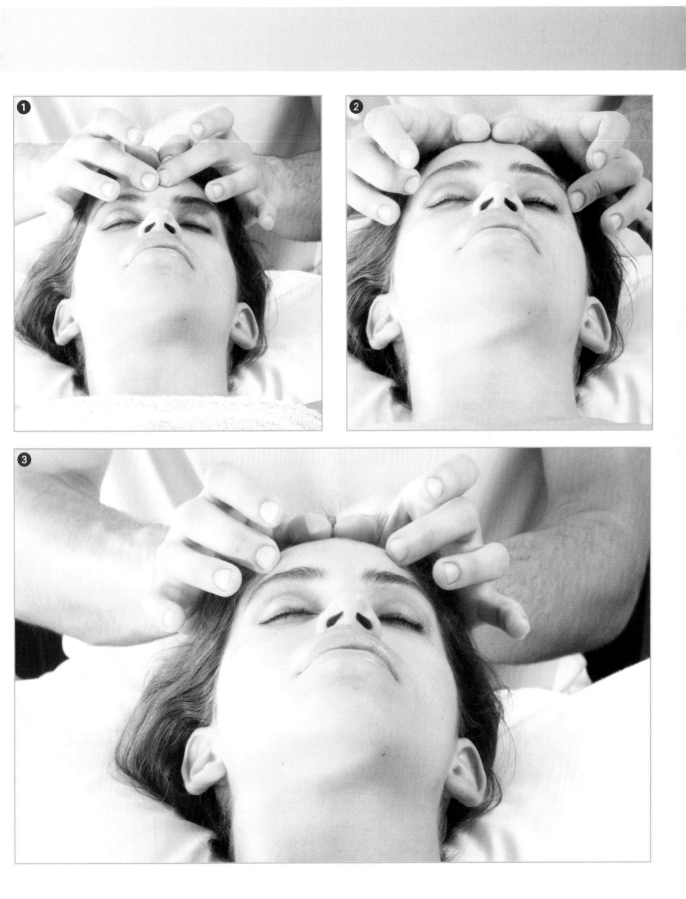

FACE (CONTINUED)

1–**2** Now place your thumbs on the forehead. Rub one thumb back and forth along one brow at a time.

CAUTION

Be sure not to place your fingers on the inside of the eye socket.

3 Next, place your middle fingers on the inside ends of the eyebrows. Glide your fingers down the bridge of the nose and around the eyes to the temples. When you reach the temple, gently massage there.

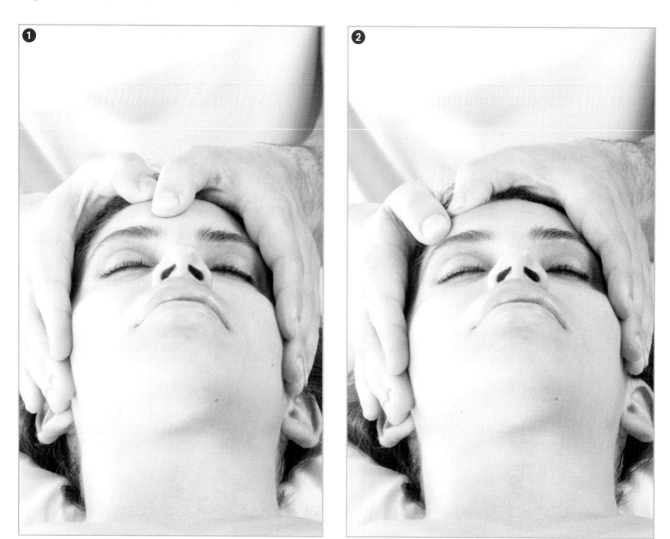

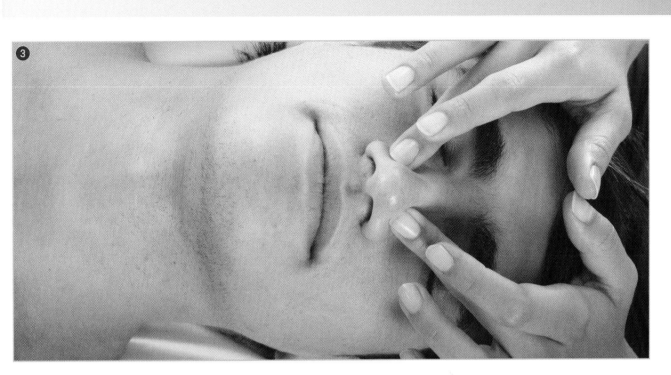

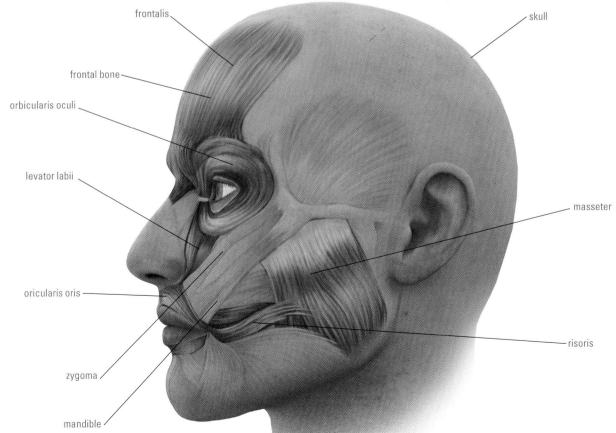

frontalis

skull

frontal bone

orbicularis oculi

levator labii

masseter

oricularis oris

risoris

zygoma

mandible

FACE (CONTINUED)

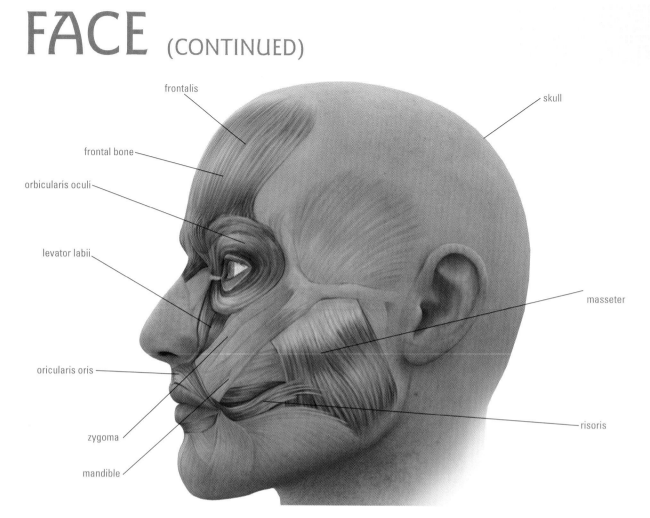

frontalis

skull

frontal bone

orbicularis oculi

levator labii

masseter

oricularis oris

zygoma

risoris

mandible

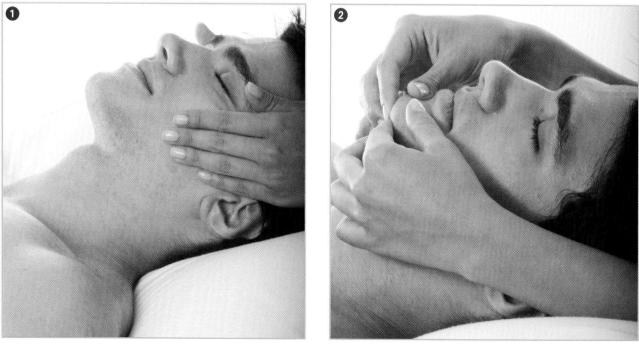

❶

❷

①–② To continue, place one hand on each side of the face and make small circles all over.

③ Next, gently squeeze the chin.

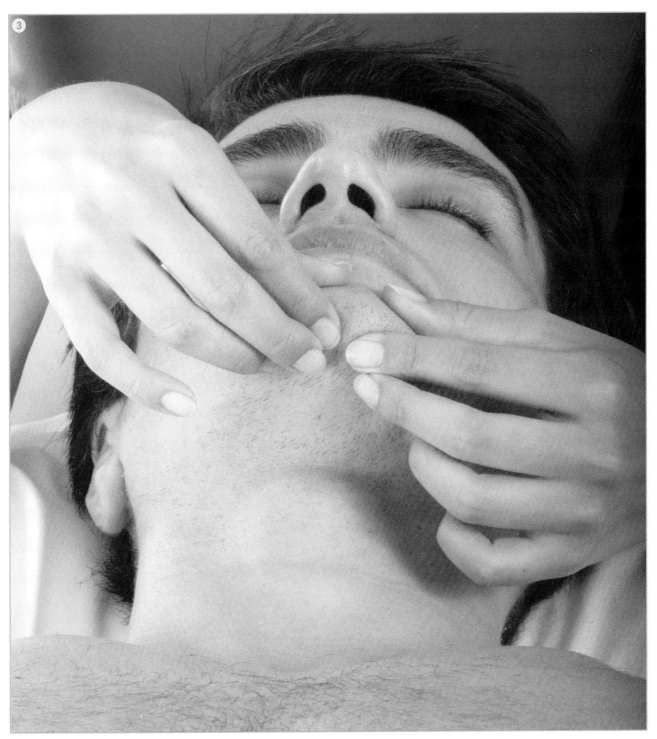

FACE (CONTINUED)

①–② Gently grasp the jaw at the chin and carefully pinch along the jawline, almost to the ear.

③ Now place your thumbs under the cheekbones and your fingers under the jaw, and massage the muscles under the chin.

Apply only very gentle pressure around the throat to avoid causing discomfort or injury.

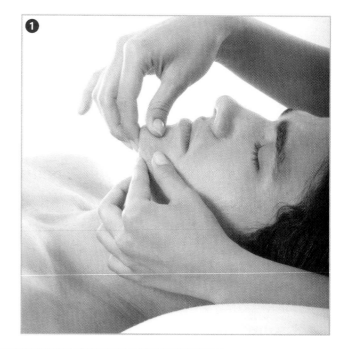

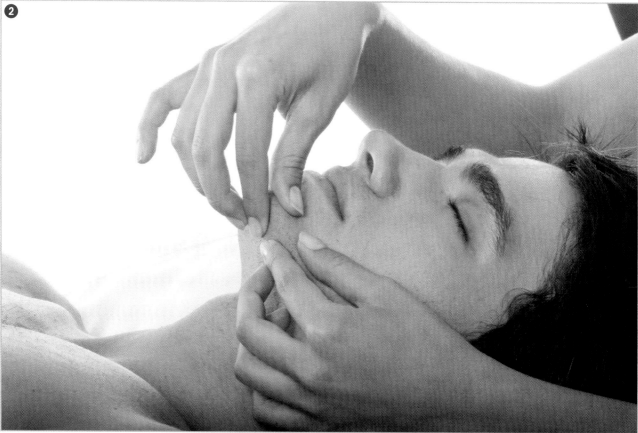

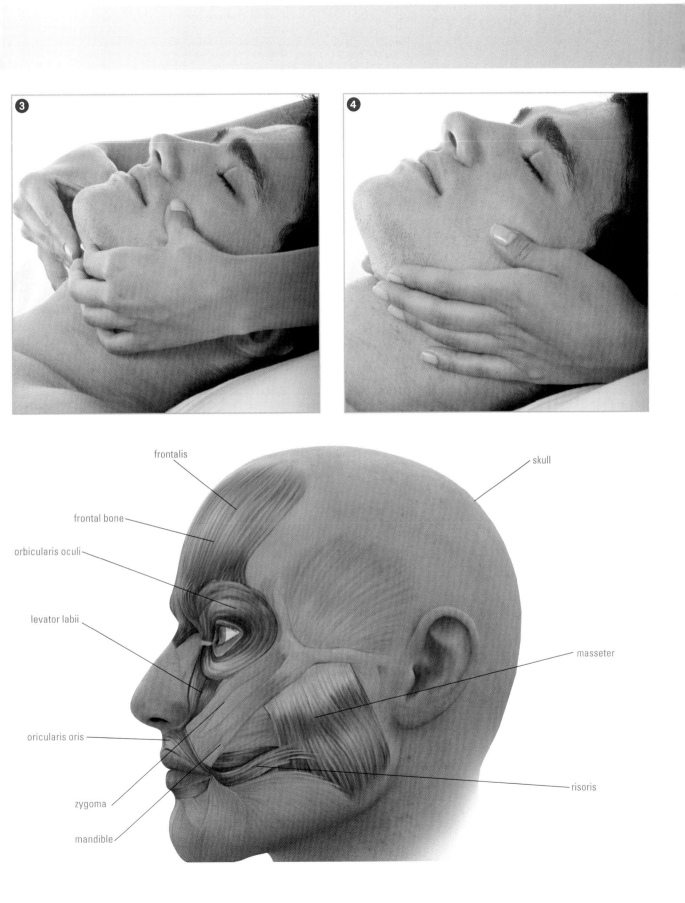

❸

❹

frontalis

skull

frontal bone

orbicularis oculi

levator labii

masseter

oricularis oris

zygoma

risoris

mandible

FACE (CONTINUED)

1 With your hands in the same position, gently stroke the face from the inside of the eye to the bottom of the cheekbone. This stroke helps to drain the sinuses.

2–**3** Next, pull your hands up the face and over the cheek.

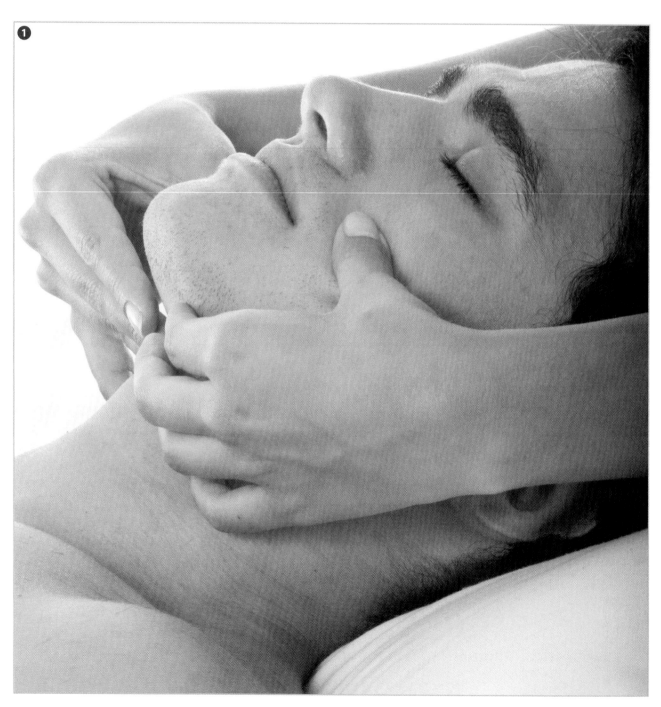

1

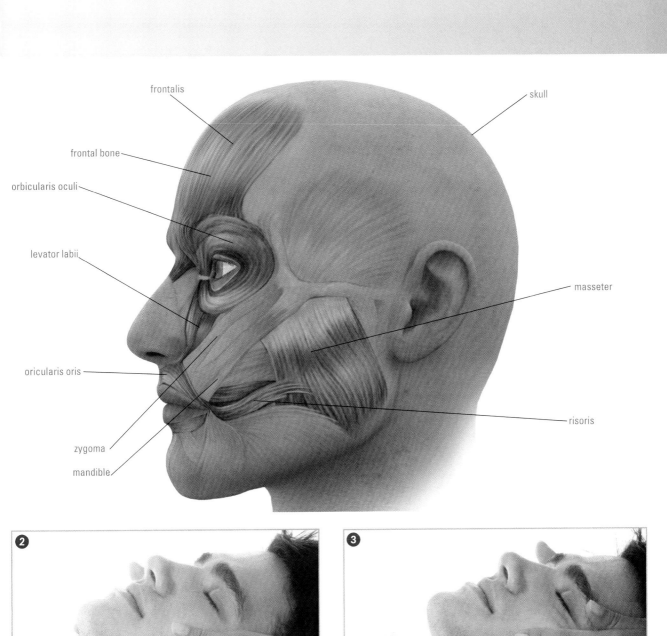

frontalis

skull

frontal bone

orbicularis oculi

levator labii

masseter

oricularis oris

zygoma

mandible

risoris

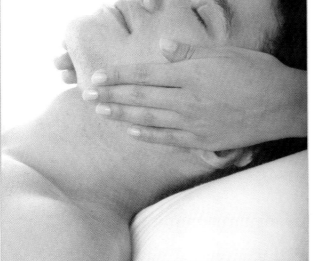

2

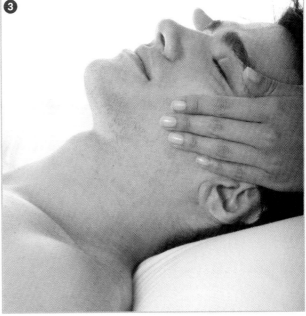

3

FACE (CONTINUED)

①–② Finish the face massage by working the earlobes. Grasp the ears and make small circles with your thumbs along the ear from the lobes to the tip.

③ Finally, grasp both earlobes and give them a gentle tug.

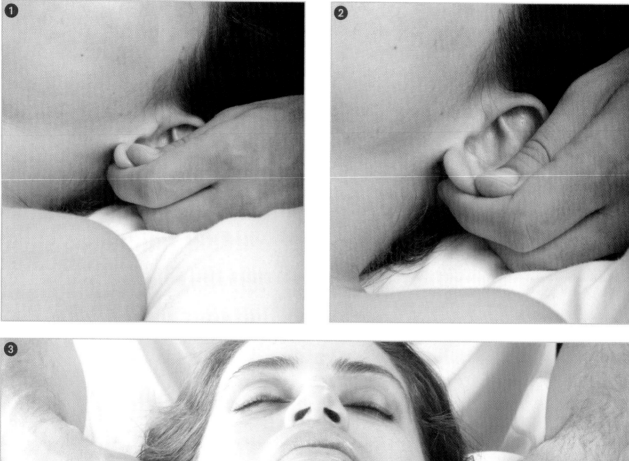

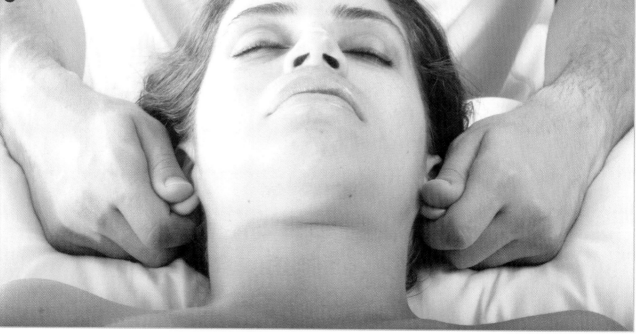

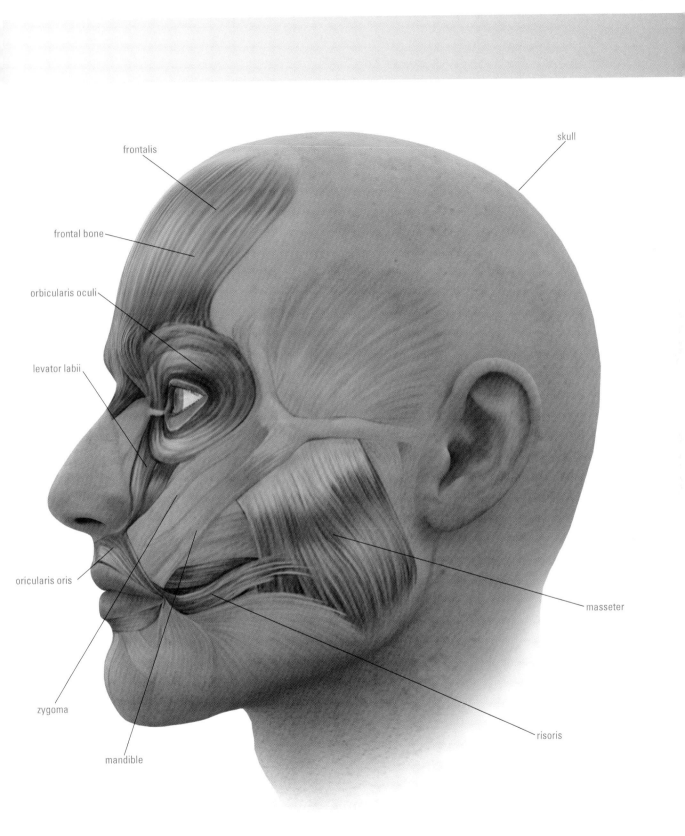

frontalis

skull

frontal bone

orbicularis oculi

levator labii

oricularis oris

masseter

zygoma

risoris

mandible

HEAD

Most of us have had our hair shampooed for us, and so we know the pleasure of a head massage. Once you have mastered the strokes of the head massage, it won't have to wait for a trip to the salon.

1–2 Place your hands on the head as shown and use your thumbs to press along a line down the center of the skull, from the widow's peak to as far back as you're able to reach comfortably.

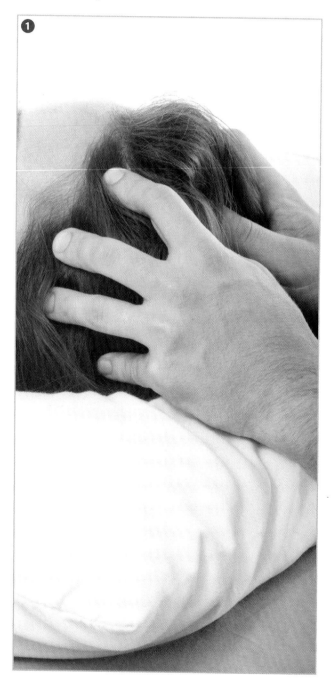

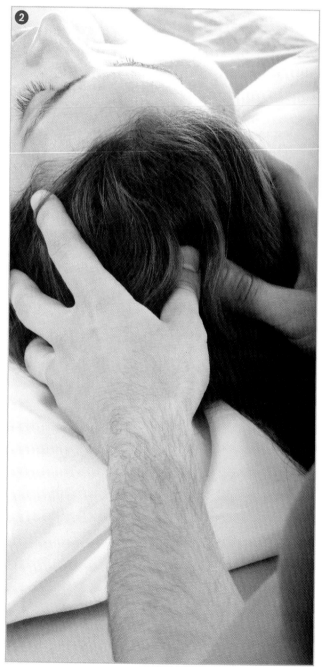

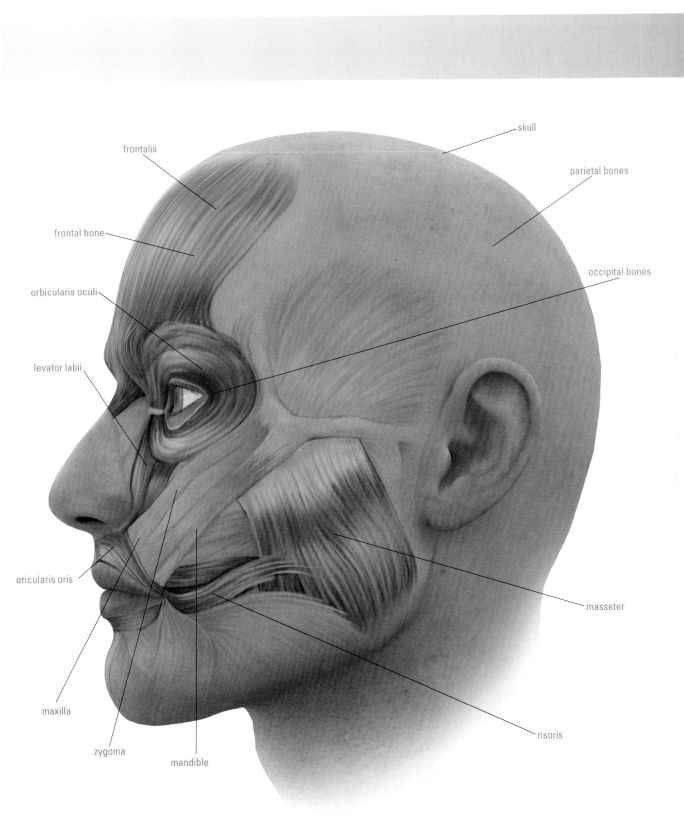

skull

parietal bones

frontalis

frontal bone

occipital bones

orbicularis oculi

levator labii

oricularis oris

masseter

maxilla

risoris

zygoma

mandible

HEAD (CONTINUED)

Finish the massage by making small circles all over the scalp, as if you were shampooing the hair.

Now that the massage is over, be mindful of the fact that the person you've been massaging is likely very relaxed. So it's not the time to flip on the lights or open the blinds. Instead, let your subject know you're finished and offer to bring him some water or tea. Give him a few minutes alone and let him sit up when he feels ready.

The person you've massaged may feel so relaxed after a long session that he may even be a little wobbly on his feet afterward. So ask him to get up slowly.

To help the relaxing effects of the massage last as long as possible, keep the room quiet. This isn't the time to engage in loud conversation or to watch a comedy. Keep all activites low-key for a few hours.

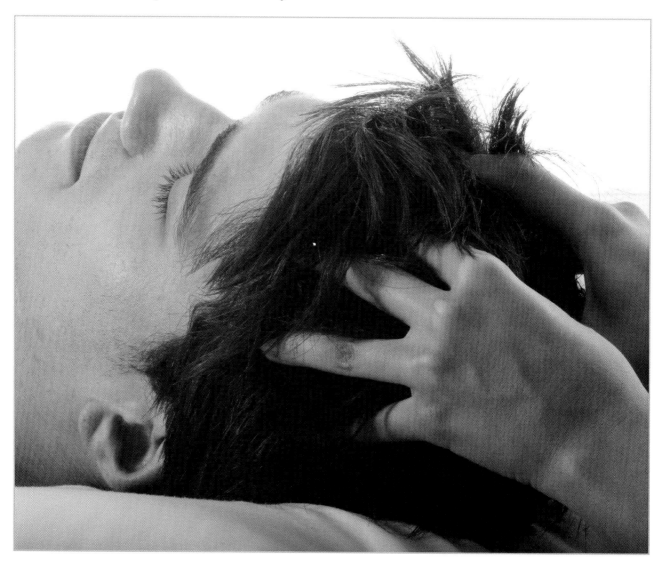

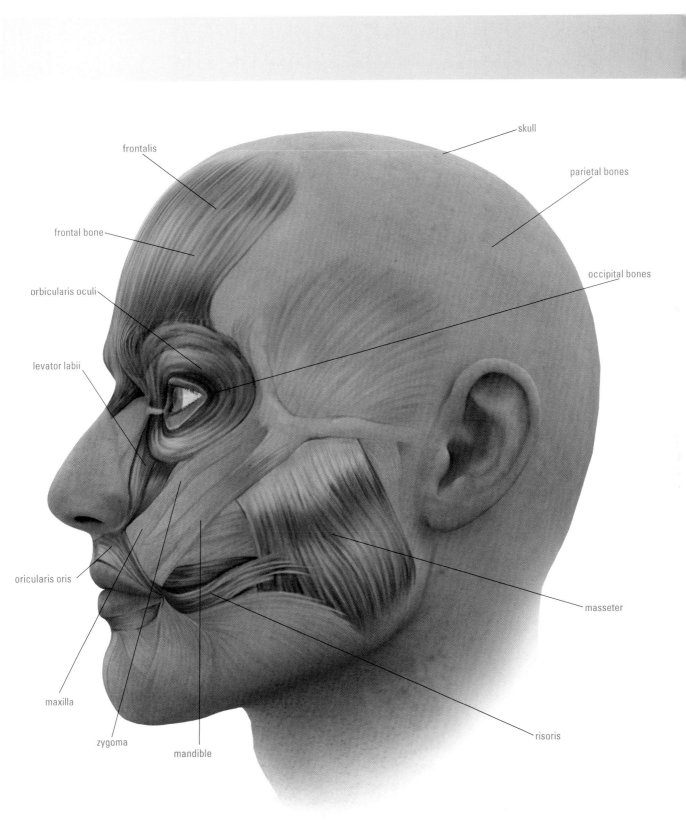

frontalis

skull

parietal bones

frontal bone

occipital bones

orbicularis oculi

levator labii

oricularis oris

masseter

maxilla

risoris

zygoma

mandible

TARGETED MASSAGES

The beauty of our massage is its versatility and adaptability. If you don't have the time for a full-body massage, you can select one of these massage sequences for a shorter, yet still invigorating, massage.

COMPUTER USER'S MASSAGE

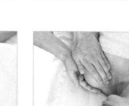

Neck (pages 130–135)

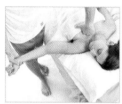
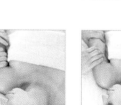

Arms & Shoulders
(pages 106–119)

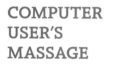

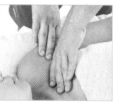
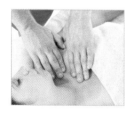
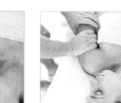
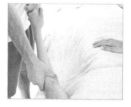

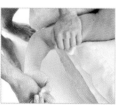
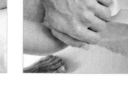
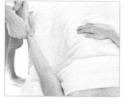
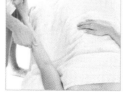
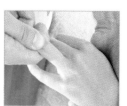

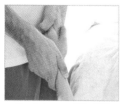
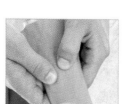
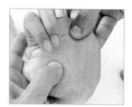
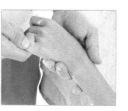

Hands (pages 120–127)

UPPER BODY TENSION RELIEF MASSAGE

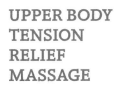
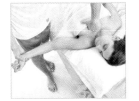
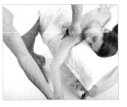
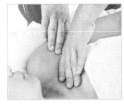
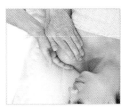

Shoulders (pages 106–117)

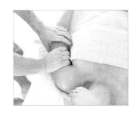
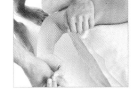
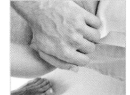
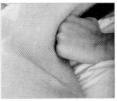
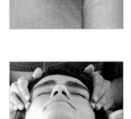

Face & Head
(pages 128–153)

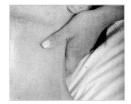
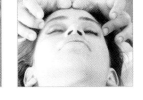
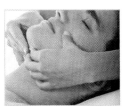
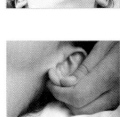
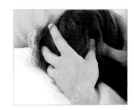

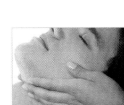
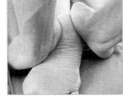
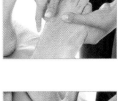

MASSAGE FOR TIRED LEGS AND FEET

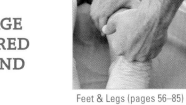

Feet & Legs (pages 56–85)

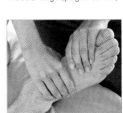
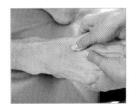
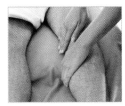
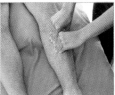

FIND OUT MORE

GLOSSARY

anterior: Located in the front.

effleurage: One of the strokes used in Swedish massage. *Effleurage*, French for "touch lightly" or "skim," is the gentle sliding stroke that relaxes the body and soft tissue before the massage begins. You'll use effleurage on each body part before massaging it.

friction: The deepest of the strokes used in Swedish massage. Friction strokes use deep, circular motions on the muscles to break down scar tissue and increase blood flow.

meridians: According to Traditional Chinese Medicine (TCM), meridians are the pathways of energy that flow through the body.

neutral position (spine): A spinal position resembling an S shape, consisting of a lordosis in the lower back, when viewed in profile.

petrissage: In Swedish massage, petrissage strokes squeeze, roll, and knead the muscles.

posterior: Located behind.

medial: Located on, or extending toward, the middle.

lateral: Located on, or extending toward, the outside.

scapula: The protrusion of bone on the mid to upper back, also known as the shoulder blade.

LATIN GLOSSARY

The following glossary explains the Latin terminology used to describe the body's musculature. Certain words are derived from the Greek, which has been indicated in each instance.

UPPER LEG

vastus lateralis: *vastus*, "immense, huge," and *lateralis*, "of the side"

vastus medialis: *vastus*, "immense, huge," and *medialis*, "middle"

vastus intermedius: *vastus*, "immense, huge," and *intermedius*, "that which is between"

rectus femoris: from *rego*, "straight, upright," and *femur*, "thigh"

adductor longus: from *adducere*, "to contract," and *longus*, "long"

adductor magnus: from *adducere*, "to contract," and *magnus*, "major"

gracilis: *gracilis*, "slim, slender"

tensor fasciae latae: from *tenere*, "to stretch," *fasciae*, "band," and *latae,* "laid down"

biceps femoris: *biceps*, "two-headed," and *femur*, "thigh"

semitendinosus: *semi*, "half," and *tendo*, "tendon"

semimembranosus: *semi*, "half," and *membrum*, "limb"

sartorius: from *sarcio*, "to patch" or "to repair"

LOWER LEG

gastrocnemii: Greek *gastroknémía*, "calf [of the leg]" and Latin suffix

soleus: *solea*, "sandal"

tibialis posterior: *tibia*, literally "reed pipe," and *posterus*, "coming after"

tibialis anterior: *tibia*, literally "reed pipe," and *ante*, "before"

peroneii: *peronei*, literally "of the fibula"

flexor hallucis: from *flectere*, "to bend," and *hallex*, "big toe"

extensor hallucis: from *extendere*, "to stretch," and *hallex*, "big toe"

HIPS

gluteus medius: Greek *gloutós*, "rump," with Latin suffix, and *medialis*, "middle"

gluteus maximus: Greek *gloutós*, "rump," with Latin suffix, and *maximus*, "largest"

gluteus minimus: Greek *gloutós*, "rump," with Latin suffix, and *minimus*, "smallest"

iliopsoas: *ilia*, variant of *ilium*, "groin," and Greek *psoa*, "groin muscle"

iliacus: *ilia*, variant of *ilium*, "groin"

obturator externus: from *obturare*, "to block," and *externus*, "outward"

obturator internus: from *obturare*, "to block," and *internus*, "within"

pectineus: *pectin*, "comb"

superior gemellus: from *super*, "above," and *geminus*, "twin"

inferior gemellus: from *inferus*, "under," and *geminus*, "twin"

piriformis: from *pirum*, "pear"; therefore "pear-shaped"

quadratus femoris: *quadratus*, "square, rectangular," and *femur*, "thigh"

TORSO

transversus abdominis: *transversus*, "athwart," and *abdomen*, "belly"

rectus abdominis: from *rego*, "straight, upright," and *abdomen*, "belly"

obliquus internus: *obliquus*, "slanting," and *internus*, "within"

obliquus externus: *obliquus*, "slanting," and *externus*, "outward"

serratus anterior: from *serra*, "saw"; therefore "saw-shaped," and *ante*, "before"

FIND OUT MORE (CONTINUED)

BACK

trapezius: Greek *trapezion*, literally "small table"

rhomboid: Greek *rhembesthai*, "to spin"

latissimus dorsi: *latus*, "wide," and *dorsum*, "back"

erector spinae: *erectus*, "straight," and *spina*, "thorn"

quadratus lumborum: *quadratus*, "square, rectangular," and *lumbus*, "loin"

CHEST

pectoralis [major and minor]: *pectus*, "breast"

coracobrachialis: Greek *korakoeidés*, "raven-like," and *brachium*, "arm"

SHOULDERS

deltoid [anterior, posterior, and medial]: Greek *deltoeidés*, "delta-shaped"

supraspinatus: *supra*, "above," and *spina*, "thorn"

infraspinatus: *infra*, "under," and *spina*, "thorn"

subscapularis: *sub*, "below," and *scapulae*, "shoulder [blades]"

teres [major and minor]: *teres*, "rounded"

levator scapulae: from *levare*, "to raise," and *scapulae*, "shoulder [blades]"

UPPER ARM

biceps brachii: *biceps*, "two-headed," and *brachium*, "arm"

triceps brachii: *triceps*, "three-headed," and *brachium*, "arm"

brachialis: *brachium*, "arm"

LOWER ARM

brachioradialis: *brachium*, "arm," and *radius*, "spoke"

extensor carpi radialis: from *extendere*, "to bend," Greek *karpós*, "wrist," and *radius*, "spoke"

flexor carpi radialis: from *flectere*, "to bend," Greek *karpós*, "wrist," and *radius*, "spoke"

extensor digitorum: from *extendere*, "to stretch," and *digitus*, "finger, toe"

flexor digitorum: from *flectere*, "to bend," and *digitus*, "finger, toe"

NECK

sternocleidomastoid: Greek *stérnon*, "chest," Greek *kleís*, "key," and Greek *mastoeidés*, "breastlike"

scalenes: Greek *skalénós*, "unequal"

splenius: Greek *splénion*, "plaster, patch"

RESOURCES

Books

Braun, Mary Beth and Stephanie J. Simonson. *Introduction to Massage Therapy*. Philadelphia: Lippincott Williams & Wilkins, 2007.

Downing, George. *The Massage Book:* 25th Anniversary Edition. New York: Random House, 1998.

Lidell, Lucinda. *The Book of Massage: The Complete Step-by-Step Guide to Eastern and Western Technique*. Fireside, 2001.

Maxwell-Hudson, Clare. *The Complete Book of Massage*. New York: Random House, 1988.

Web Sites

American Massage Therapy Association
http://www.amtamassage.org/
Professional association for massage therapists; features extensive information about massage for consumers

Best Massage
http://www.bestmassage.com
Portable and stationary massage tables; accessories including massage table covers, bolsters and supports, DVDs, books, and music

Core Products
http://www.coreproducts.com
Massage cushions, bolsters, and oil and lotion holsters

Gaiam
http://www.gaiam.com
Clothing, supplies, and resources for massage, yoga, and fitness

Massage King
http://www.massageking.com
Massage tables for home users; gifts and accessory kits

Massage Warehouse
http://www.massagewarehouse.com
Features a wide variety of massage products—especially aromatherapy products (essential oils and blends, mists and sprays, candles), massage equipment (tables and chairs, table accessories, tools), and music

OmStream
http://www.omstream.com
Downloadable music for massage and yoga

One Touch Massage
http://www.1massagestore.com
Massage furniture (massage tables, bolster pillows, sheets and linens, chairs, and stools) as well as tools and supplies (lotions and oils)

Pristine Planet
http://www.pristineplanet.com
Eco-friendly natural and organic massage oils

Scandle
http://www.abodycandle.com
Soy candles in a variety of scents that melt into massage oil

Sequoia Records
http://www.sequoiarecords.com
Music for meditation, yoga, spa, and relaxation

CREDITS & ACKNOWLEDGMENTS

All photos by Jonathan Conklin/Jonathan Conklin Photography except for the following pages:

8 vnlit/Shutterstock **9** Matt Antonino/Shutterstock
11 Night and Day Images/Shutterstock **11** Jerko
Grubisic/Shutterstock **13** Gunnar Pippel/Shutterstock
15 Igumnova Irina/Shutterstock **15** viviamo/Shutterstock
16 GG.Image/Shutterstock **61** Perkus/Shutterstock
87 Wolfgang Amri/Shutterstock **108** Anatoly Khudobin

Models: Monica Ordonez and Roland Szegi

All illustrations by Hector Aiza/3D Labz Animation India

ACKNOWLEDGMENTS

The author and publisher offer thanks to those closely
involved in the creation of this book: Moseley Road
president Sean Moore; editor Lori Baird; editorial director
Lisa Purcell; art director Brian MacMullen; designers
Holly Lee and Neil Dvorak; and assistant editor Jon
Derengowski.